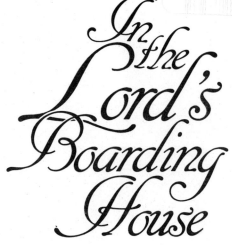

In the Lord's Boarding House

To my parents

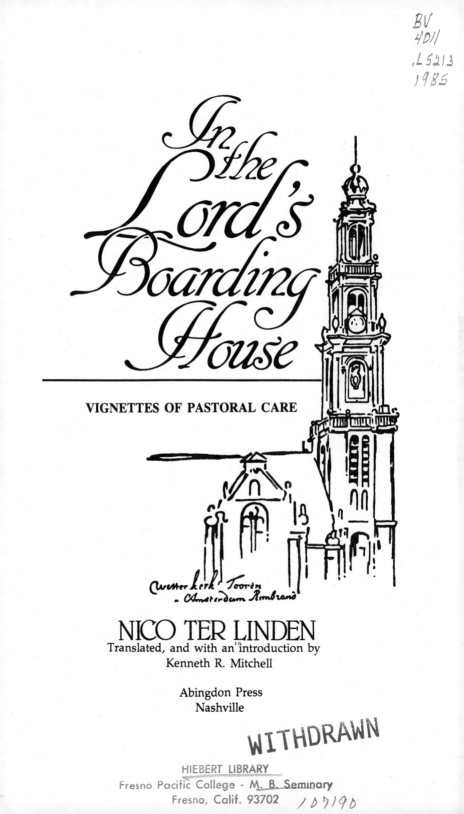

In the Lord's Boarding House

VIGNETTES OF PASTORAL CARE

Westerkerk Tooren
- Amsterdam Rembrand

NICO TER LINDEN

Translated, and with an introduction by
Kenneth R. Mitchell

Abingdon Press
Nashville

In the Lord's Boarding House

Translation copyright © 1985 by Abingdon Press

Library of Congress Cataloging in Publication Data

Linden, Nico ter.
  In the Lord's boarding house.
  Translation of: Lieve landgenoten and Kostgangers.
  1. Pastoral theology—Addresses, essays, lectures.
2. Clergy—Office—Addresses, essays, lectures.
I. Linden, Nico ter. Kostgangers. English. 1985. II. Title.
BV4011.L5213 1985   253'.092'6   84-24545

ISBN 0-687-18971-3

© 1979—Gooi en Sticht bv, Hilversum, Holland: Lieve landgenoten

© 1981—Gooi en Sticht bv, Hilversum, Holland: Kostgangers

Scripture quotations noted RSV are taken from the Revised Standard Version of the Bible, copyrighted 1946, 1952, © 1971, 1973.

Lines from *The Threepenny Opera* from *Bertolt Brecht: Collected Plays*, vol. 2, ed. Ralph Manheim and John Willett (New York: Vintage Books, 1977), pp. 164-65.

All other quotations and scripture quotations are translated from the Dutch.

Manufactured by the Parthenon Press at
Nashville, Tennessee, United States of America

Contents

Introduction...7

All Ears..13

Gratitude...15

The Lord Is My Shepherd............................ 17

The Lord Is *Not* My Shepherd...................... 20

Doubt...22

Polarization... 24

Boxing... 27

Praying for the Neighbor............................29

Blessing.. 32

Something...37

Body and Soul... 39

Do-It-Yourselfer..42

Punishment.. 44

Jabbok... 46

Dying.. 49

Tolerance... 55

Cross-Eyed Angels..................................... 57

Anticipation..62

Dreaming.. 65

Panizza.. 67

Francis...70

Pain...73

Gary Gilmore...75

Senile.. 77

Breath..80

Millstone.. 83

Weary Wanderer.. 86

A Little Pastoral Word List...........................88

Faith Stories... 94

Hospitable Church......................................97

Cemetery..101
Mourning.. 103
Hoping and Wishing...................................105
Morning Blessing.......................................107
Calling... 110
Questions.. 113
Looking..116
Born of God...119
Gerard...121
The Old Wester Tower............................... 124

Introduction

Nico ter Linden has "waited on table" in many versions of the Lord's boarding house: a village in the province of North Holland, a small Reformed parish in an otherwise Catholic town in the Catholic province of North Brabant, prisons in Kansas and in two towns in the Netherlands, medical and psychiatric clinics, and now in one of the great Dutch churches, the Westerkerk in Amsterdam.

I first met Dominee ter Linden while he was pastor of the little Reformed Church in Lith, a village on the banks of the busy Maas River. At the same time, he was a graduate student at the Catholic University of Nijmegen, where I was serving as visiting professor of pastoral psychology for a semester. Father Willy Zandbelt and I jointly supervised a group of doctoral students who brought their experiences in ministry for review by their teachers and their peers. Even my somewhat inexperienced ear for the Dutch language could catch the difference when ter Linden spoke; his intelligence and his imagination produced speech that was eloquent, earthy, and vivid. That made me work hard, but it was a pleasure to deepen and broaden my Dutch so that I could grasp more clearly what Dominee ter Linden was saying.

I later had the privilege of having him as a student in the Division of Religion and Psychiatry at the Menninger Foundation, where I was then working. He came to Kansas for a year with his wife, Annette, and their three children. Shortly after their return to the Netherlands and the completion of his work in Nijmegen, he was called to the pulpit of the Westerkerk, the historic church near the Anne Frank house.

The Westerkerk stands by the Prinsengracht or Prince's Canal, one of the great waterways that ring (and define) the center of Amsterdam. In front of this beautiful old church stands "its" tower, the Westertoren. (The word *its* has to be in quotation marks, because the church building belongs to the Westerkerk congregation, but the tower is the property of the city of Amsterdam.) Next to the church is a marketplace in use in the time of Rembrandt, who is buried in the church. On the other side of the canal is the Jordaan, a blue-collar residential district whose inhabitants celebrate life and death and the Wester Tower in song.

The Wester is one of the great churches of the city; unlike some of the others, it has a lively congregational life. You can, as Dominee ter Linden says, listen to a Bach Festival in the church in the morning, and then cross the canal to a café where you will hear the songs of the Jordaan with accordion accompaniment. You will see some of the same people in both places.

The layout of the church might strike you as odd. Like the sanctuary in many American churches, the Wester's is relatively long and narrow. But the "preekstoel" or pulpit stands halfway along one side of the church. The congregation faces to the "side." Above them, in a gallery to their left over the front door and the vestibule, is the organ console. Though the organ's air is now supplied by electric motors, it is possible to step behind the console into a small chamber and see the great treadles once operated by the organist's assistants, who trod out the air while hanging on to a brass pole which looks as if it belongs in a fire station.

On Palm Sunday in 1979, Nico ter Linden sent me a copy of a little book called *Lieve Landgenoten*. The title means "Dear Compatriots," a phrase with powerful meaning for the Dutch, whose Queen Wilhelmina began her broadcasts to her people from exile in England during World War II with those words. Choosing one of the essays ("Senile") at random, I found that I was reading an unusually sensitive story about ministry. I made a quick translation for one of my classes at Eden Seminary; the students and I both found it powerful. I sought and received Dominee ter Linden's permission to translate the whole book and submit it to an American publisher. Since then, Dominee ter Linden has published two more volumes of essays: *Kostgangers* (from which the title of this English translation is taken) and *Schoffelen in de Wijngaard* (Hoeing in the Vineyard). Most of the essays originally appeared in Dominee ter Linden's column "Lieve Landgenoten," published in *Hervormd Nederland*, a magazine of the Dutch

Reformed Church. Some were originally the scripts of television presentations.

Boarding house? An unusual symbol for the church, drawn from a Dutch saying. If you're walking down the street or sitting in a sidewalk café somewhere in the Netherlands, you may see an unusual person pass by: an odd gait, strange clothing, a striking face. And your Dutch companion might well say, *"Onze Lieve Heer heeft rare kostgangers"* (Our Dear Lord keeps strange boarders at his table). The comment may be made with disdain or affection. Just right as an image of the church.

★　★　★

Short essays of the kind to be found in this book are almost a Dutch specialty. Perhaps that is because the country itself is small: one-fifth the size of the state of Missouri, a little larger than Maryland. Some of the best Dutch writers of recent years—Godfried Bomans, Simon Carmiggelt—have chosen the "miniature" or short essay as their preferred form. When the Dutch paint on small canvases, they manage somehow to convey a wealth of detail. They are often content to show one small facet of human life, knowing that their work is somehow a holograph; human life as a whole is illuminated by it. So it often is with painters such as Vermeer, and so it is with writers such as Carmiggelt or Bomans—or with this book.

A conversation with a church elder about cemeteries illuminates the problems of taking people just as they are and serving them in the name of Christ. A young prisoner's fanciful dreaming about a nonexistent inheritance becomes the springboard for a new understanding of the meaning of Easter. The clinch in a boxing match tells us something about what happened to Patty Hearst. Ter Linden wrote the essays for people in his own country and his own church, and sometimes they are very Dutch; yet Americans will recognize themselves and their own situation repeatedly. The author wrote for the church at large, and not just for pastors; but pastors will find rich resources for pastoral care in these glimpses of parish, prison, and hospital.

★　★　★

Some idioms are difficult to translate from one language to another; others are simply impossible. The more the original writer is a master of the craft of writing, the more the images are unique and colorful, and thus the more difficult to convey in another language.

Some Dutch idioms have distinct English counterparts. In "The Lord Is My Shepherd," an old woman is quoted as saying, "I've got a bone to pick with God." What she actually said was, "I've got an apple to peel with God." We pick bones while the Dutch peel apples; in either case it is not too difficult to convey the underlying meaning of the phrase.

There are other thoughts and ideas which simply cannot be brought into another language as deftly as they were originally put. In "Morning Blessing," the use of the name of one city—Paramaribo—immediately conveys to a Dutch reader a collection of images and bits of history. From that one word, and from almost no other evidence, ter Linden's Dutch readers knew that the woman asking for a blessing was black. More than that, they were aware of the mixed feelings aroused in the Netherlands when many people from Paramaribo, most of them black, emigrated to Europe while Surinam (formerly Dutch Guiana, with Paramaribo as its capital) was still a province of the European Netherlands, before it received its independence. The influx of these fellow countrymen who somehow were also not fellow countrymen confronted the Dutch with racial problems they had previously been able to deny. In the original text no mention is made of the fact that the woman was black; I felt it necessary to insert that identification near the beginning so that American readers would understand more clearly what ter Linden was dealing with as a pastor.

Add to that his own memories of the terrible "hunger winter" near the end of World War II—starvation, land mines, barbed wire—and the fact that this pastoral work with the woman from Paramaribo took him back to an area of the city that held vivid and painful memories for him, and was now a minority ghetto. Translating an essay such as "Morning Blessing" is a challenging intellectual puzzle, and at the same time a deeply moving experience. It is also a frustration, for the translator cannot help knowing that he is merely scratching the surface. No translation will ever convey all the richness of the original; I am sure that I am not even aware of all the richness of the original. I am particularly grateful for the help of the author himself and his friends, English teachers Piet and Ria Schipper. (But of course they are not responsible for any mistakes.) The limitations of translation do not rob the book of its warmth or its underlying strengths.

★ ★ ★

Among those strengths is the contribution Dominee ter Linden makes to pastoral care and pastoral theology.

His time at the Menninger Foundation took place when pastoral care was struggling with an issue. Modern pastoral care began with the work of the Reverend Anton T. Boisen, who insisted that beginning pastors must study "living human documents." As his students did so, and their students, they became more and more interested in psychology and sociology. It was natural and even welcome that they should have done that; psychology, and in particular the dynamic psychology of the early twentieth century, seemed to offer a way of understanding human beings that deeply enriched pastoral care.

But that enrichment came at the price of pastors neglecting their theology. Theology had previously been used so defensively that supervisors of clinical pastoral education—the heirs of Boisen—assumed that *every* reference to theology was defensive. Meanwhile, the insights of psychology proved so powerful that *only* psychological talk seemed to make sense when discussing the problems of human beings. A few leaders—Seward Hiltner, Wayne Oates, and the late Thomas W. Klink among them—insisted that we had to retain and recover our theological roots. Under Klink's leadership, the staff of the Division of Religion and Psychiatry at the Menninger Foundation was determined to work at that task. I joined the staff for precisely that purpose. We were strongly supported by Paul W. Pruyser, at that time the Director of the

Foundation's Department of Education. Pruyser, a native of the Netherlands, is a clinical psychologist with a deep interest in theology, and a Presbyterian elder. In his work with the Division of Religion and Psychiatry, as in his books, Pruyser insisted that ministers recapture their own rightful place as theologians.

This was the milieu into which Nico ter Linden stepped when he came to this country to study. It nurtured him and added to his own already strong psychological and theological interests. The result is a collection of pieces that makes a major contribution to the work of pastors and to the understanding of pastoral care.

Thinking about one's work from both psychological and theological perspectives is like looking at things through a pair of glasses with one lens tinted green and the other red. The two eyes do not notice the same things. The difference between what one sees through the green lens and what one sees through the red lens is at first confusing but in the long run enriching.

So it is with ter Linden's writing. The same objects are there in both cases, but are seen from different vantage points. The interplay between the two differing ways of looking at human situations is capable of keeping the pastor a pastor while at the same time enriching pastoral work immeasurably. That is what Nico ter Linden has done in this book. We are in his debt.

All Ears

He couldn't get along without his wife, but he couldn't get along *with* her, either; and when he got drunk, his emotional brakes quickly failed, and he'd hit her.

In the detention center we called men like him *commuters*: the police regularly came to bring him in for a few months.

He was a faithful member of our discussion group. "Chaplain, I want to ask you something: do you have a call? And then I've got another question: that fairy tale about Adam and Eve in paradise, do you believe that?"

I answered him. About a call I'd had an evasive but acceptable lecture for years, so that was no problem. And I can give a good lecture about the Creation story, and a very instructive one, at that.

So it irritated me a bit that, after he'd come back from a few months away, he came up with his question again: "Chaplain, let me ask you something: do you have a call? And then, too: that story about Adam and Eve in paradise, you believe that?"

Patiently I repeated my wisdom, in the hope that this time he'd listen better.

★   ★   ★

Only later did it dawn on me that it was I who had to learn to listen. "What's the man asking?" said my supervisor. I restated the questions. "Yes, those are his words, but why does this man ask these questions?" I didn't know. But my supervisor thought he knew. "Want to bet?" he said.

A month or so later our client was back in the pokey. We greeted each other as old acquaintances. I wasn't at all surprised—really, I was kind of glad—when he promptly came up with his questions again, whether I had a call and whether I thought the story of Adam and Eve a fairy tale. So I said to him: "If I get your drift, you're wondering whether there *is* a God who calls people. You're wondering if I've had any experience of that, because you haven't—you seriously doubt that God is calling to you and if you and your Eve might ever be happy again as a couple or if you can just forget that paradise story. Is that what you mean?"

"Yes," he said, "That's what I want to know."

Well, why had I listened so poorly before? Why had I translated so inadequately my calling into his, that happy couple from the past into this unhappy couple of the present? First of all, lack of skill, but more than that: lack of faith. Let me honestly confess that I really didn't believe at all that things could work out well for this man and for his marriage. All I saw was a heap of ruins, and faith always sees farther than that. But I didn't see it. And I didn't listen. That man posed insoluble problems for me, and I lacked the courage to accompany him all the way to the end of his painful path.

In such a case listening means sharing pain, and I didn't have enough faith in the house to take up that cross. Then I had to learn something that I have to learn over and over again, because my belief keeps having to struggle with my unbelief. I have to learn (to use the words of an American pastor) that whoever is not prepared to descend into hell with another cannot ascend into heaven with him.

★ ★ ★

I got a letter from an old man who'd just paid a visit to his brother, who in turn had confided to him that he was remembering things more and more poorly.

"My head is just like a sieve, and it's getting worse all the time," the brother had said. And the old man had answered, "Yes, old age brings infirmities."

It was only on the way home on the train that he'd realized what a conversation-stopper that had been. "I should have said something like 'I think you're terribly anxious that soon you won't be able to have a real conversation with your wife and kids.' Then my brother would probably have felt understood, and I'd have been closer to him, right where he's afraid of being, in his isolation."

Listening is hard because it costs so much and we aren't always ready to pay the price. To try to surrender yourself to hearing words, and the words behind the words which reveal how another thinks and feels, is something you do out of trust, in the hope that you'll come out somewhere near where the Lord is, but you're never sure you get there. It has to do with wanting to save your life or being willing to lose it. One must pay a high price to become all ears. The seed must die in order to bear fruit.

And that's hard.

Gratitude

I don't believe I've ever met a lonelier person. Her songs of woe in the sickroom knew no end, and just when they were ready to release her and send her home, she teased her wounds open on the sly with a knitting needle, and so the lamentations began all over again.

In the summer she was allowed to take a week's trip on a Red Cross excursion steamer, the *Henri Dunant*. Then she'd send herself, ahead of time, postcards at the various ports of call: "Love from Aunt Lucy," "Greetings from the Binkhorst family," and whoever else might arise in her fantasy. The cards were stuck on the wall above her bed, bizarre evidence of just-look-at-all-the-people-who-think-of-me. There was no one who thought of her with any warmth. "But, I'm a praying woman, remember," she said. "I pray. Every morning I say, 'Lord, here is your handmaiden.' And after that I always say, 'The mess is beginning again!' "

From time to time I have to think of her, because I hear her pained, offended tones every day on all the radio stations, and it costs me now, just as it did then, the greatest effort to keep listening with love. It's a puzzle to me how they get those soured people in front of the microphone or the camera to grumble and gripe about everything from left to right that doesn't please them, chilly songs of woe about their troubles and about being left out in the cold, discriminated against, duped, hassled, shut out.

Now, not being satisfied with the world is a good Christian virtue, and you'll never hear me say that they're wrong, but *un*satisfied people are a different kettle of fish from *dis*satisfied people—and what wears me out and makes me suspicious is that so many who are "fighting for freedom" are themselves so unfree.

How inconvenient it'll be for you if the kingdom comes tomorrow, I find myself thinking. (I don't always have myself well in hand, and particularly not in the early morning, when I'm driving to work and have to listen to all that garbage on my car radio.)

The morning devotions on the radio are mostly not fit for human consumption. (I think those speakers should be compelled to write their brilliant scripts at the same ungodly hour when we believers have to listen to it all.) *The mess is beginning all over again*, I say to myself. I turn the knob and try to give myself some quiet time, all the while trying not to let the birds of the air and the flowers of the field out of my vision. They toil not, neither do they sow, but our heavenly Father feeds them anyhow. Often I see, in my mind's eye, the black preacher in Kansas City. Reverently and boisterously we were celebrating the kingdom of God on a Sunday morning, and then it got quite still, and he stood up and said: "God, I thank you for this day, a day we have never seen before."

What he prayed after that I haven't the least idea, for I'd had enough already. A simpler prayer is hardly imaginable, but it was such a stunning thing for me, and it's often helped me since then to open my eyes—really open them—in the morning and to say, full of gratitude and wonder: "My Lord, what a morning!"

"Gratitude," said the old pastor in our village, "is a little plant that I fear will soon no longer bloom in any garden." If he's right, that's too bad for grace. For anyone who doesn't know gratitude, in whose garden that flower doesn't bloom (because it's never been planted or watered), grace is just excess baggage. And if pretty soon all that's left is people who have their rights, then God's going to be left sitting with a whole batch of unused grace on his hands.

Who really pays attention to grace in our day? Preachers on the early morning devotions—but that's their stock in trade. And fighting schoolboys who in our country yell "grace" the way American kids yell "uncle" or "I give." And not another soul. We have little conception left of God's gracious lordship over the world. We don't want to be dependent on grace; we have our *rights*. We want nothing from grace; a gracious God seems as archaic as a German calling a woman "gracious Lady." Like that kind of behavior, grace seems right out of the nineteenth century. In Dutch law courts people can ask for "grace from the Queen," but in the world of justice and law courts we also see the tendency to encase the right to grace in *laws*, so that the concept no longer has any relevance in our society.

We've lost something, but we've gained something, too. When they used to talk about gratitude in the family, they usually meant that children were to be subservient to their parents. The poor, the widows, the unemployed: they no longer have to be grateful for gifts; they have their rights. They no longer eat the bread of grace, the crumbs from the tables of the rich. They have rights, and they don't have to say "thank you" to anybody.

And yet. People who don't have to say "thank you" to anybody are often very unhappy people. "People who need people are the luckiest people in the world," sings Barbra Streisand. They experience grace and can be gracious. They know about messes that start all over again, but they look at them with different eyes, and, as dawn breaks in the East, they see it as a highly original day of creation by our Lord.

The Lord Is My Shepherd

She lived with a bunch of dogs and cats on a raggedy farm in a back corner of the county. Her life story was a bad novel. Her father and her husband left this life one after the other, after being kicked by a horse, and she remained behind, childless. Stubbornly she wanted to keep the farm going. But she became filthy; the land became a wasteland; people avoided her, and they had their reasons. When she could no longer make the payments on her mortgage, the bailiff came and literally and figuratively put her out in the cold. Bankrupt.

We found a nice little house for her but speculated that she wouldn't live there long. "You mustn't be surprised if you hear that I've drowned myself," she said. She looked at the drainage ditch in front of the house, and I told her that she'd do well to look for deeper water than that. "Shame on you!" she said. "You shouldn't be talking like that." I asked her what I *should* be saying. Well, she said, that life is a gift from God and that you have to deal faithfully with it. And a lot more. I found it a nice sermon, and so did she.

She was one of those strange boarders our Lord keeps at his table, somebody with a "difficult character," as they put it in the village, but in any case someone with character, and she had more depths in her little finger than many of those who shunned her had in their whole bodies. She lived close to God. They didn't understand that very well in the village; there the idea was that living close to God meant living quite well.

Just once I saw her in church. A handful of us were sitting there singing, and then in she came in a tattered coat, wearing a crazy hat. She sat down without a hymnbook, but I thought, come on now, you know that hymn perfectly well—and sure enough, after a couple of lines she got it, and then she sang and made a face at the pulpit, and I winked back. A picture, that old hermit lady at the Lord's table, to which people may come and eat and drink not because they are good but because God is good. I decided to read the psalm I'd read when we buried her mother a few years earlier: Psalm 23. I saw that she had to cry a little.

She wound up in a hospital, a Catholic hospital, and that was a good joke played by our Lord, for she'd been taught from her youth up that Catholics were no good.

She lay alone in a room, and when I asked if she could stick it out, she nodded and flicked her eyes at the wall, where a crucifix was hanging. "My Savior," she said, and somehow that sounded good and Protestant.

"I'll see you in three weeks," I said. "I'm going on vacation."

"Well, then, we won't see each other again," she said, "because I'm dying. Will you read Psalm 23 with me?"

For Protestants, reading that psalm is a bit like the last rites for Catholics, and I shrank back. I didn't want any part of it, no death in my life, thank you. I sputtered and mumbled something like "never say die" and all the other things a frightened person says, and I didn't have my Bible with me—and suddenly she herself sang the song, stubborn to the end, and I just sang along: "The Lord is my shepherd, I shall not want." *How can you sing that,* I thought, *when you do want?*

A few days later she was dead.

★ ★ ★

"What's dying like?" asked our six-year old son.

"You go to sleep and you don't wake up," I said, polishing up the awful reality a bit.

When I came back late that night from the funeral, the boy was still awake. "You'd better go to him for a bit," said my wife. "I don't know what's going on, but he can't sleep." The little one didn't dare let the day out of his hands, couldn't entrust himself to the night. I laid my hand on his head. "Go on to sleep now, see you tomorrow," I said. Then he went to sleep. He had my blessing.

★ ★ ★

This is the story of an old woman, a young man, and a child. A story of belief and unbelief.

The little one believed. Father is my shepherd, my father can do anything, he is almighty, I fear no evil, even though I go through the valley of the shadow of death—see you tomorrow.

But a boy becomes a man, loses his father, and faith comes under attack. "The Savior" is no longer or not yet "*my* Savior." Your life gets kicked in the shins, night without end. Faith, so self-evident for a child who experiences basic security with mother and father, can go bankrupt as goodness and mercy are replaced by evil. The Lord is *not* my shepherd.

But there are people—and sometimes I think you have to grow old to become one of them—who can yield up the day, or their lives, out of their hands in a faith and trust that recalls the faith and trust of a child. The only difference is that the child has never faced the possibility of unbelief.

There are those who say that it's all imagination that there's a father who waits for you at the end of the night. That may be so. It may also be the case that that absurd thought is no dream, but a well grounded expectation that God will turn out to be almighty after all.

I think that was the faith of that woman. She didn't deliver herself sheepishly into the hands of the shepherd. I've had a difficult life, she said. It all turned out very differently from what I'd hoped or expected. I wouldn't wish my life on anybody. But it was my life, just the same, it belonged to me, and I lived it. I certainly have a bone to pick with God, and he probably has a bone to pick with me, but that's all right. The Lord is my shepherd. And now I'll go to sleep.

The Lord Is **Not** *My Shepherd*

My grandfather was a minister. If anyone told him that he'd preached a good sermon, he used to reply immediately that the devil had already told him that.

Sharper still was the reaction of the chaplain in the American prison where I worked. When a swindler, tears in his eyes, would stammer, "Thank you, Chaplain, that was good," he'd get a clap on the shoulders and a hearty "What do you mean it was good? It was excellent!" And they'd remain good friends.

I myself got positive reactions to an evening devotion I did on television entitled "The Lord Is My Shepherd." And I usually don't know exactly what to say. This time, however, I asked a couple of people if it wouldn't be too immodest of me to ask what they'd found good about it. The answers were astonishing, for in many cases people seemed to be most taken by my acknowledgment that it is possible that the Lord is *not* our shepherd.

I'd said that of course it's possible, as some people insist, that the wish is father to the thought. In a shepherdless world where we just drudge along like orphans in the shadow of death, we dream of an almighty Father who holds this world and its inhabitants in his hand. Could it be true? I think it's true, but most of my friends believe nothing of the sort, and sometimes I'm not at all sure which of us is crazy. But we seem to have gotten closer together when I suggested the possibility that the

Lord is in fact not our shepherd. The expression of that thought had done many people good. I found that amazing.

But, after all, that's nonsense. For as far as I can figure out, my own belief is far more formed by people of little faith than by people of great faith. I've gotten more from seekers than from those unwavering souls who are sure that they stand on solid rock. To put it another way, my faith is, as I see it, not so much formed by the faith of others as by their struggles with faith. I want to tell you a story about that which is important for me.

There were eight of us prison chaplains—four Protestant ministers and four Catholic priests—listening to a tape recording of a sermon by one of the Catholic chaplains about probation, a sermon given in a parish somewhere. Its theme: mercy toward prisoners. It was a beautiful sermon, and so said we all. But at the end a young priest who was our guest that day had a word to say. He said, "I take it that you're saying that we must be merciful toward prisoners, is that right?" "Right," came the answer. "And you think I should want to do that?"

"Don't you?" asked the chaplain who had preached the sermon. The young priest hesitated. "No," he said. "I don't believe I want to. . . . I . . . I think I don't have much faith."

Here we go again, I thought, *another priest who's fallen away from his faith,* and I was about to haul a supportive word out of my treasury of good advice when our teacher joined him by saying, "Neither do I." Four distraught ministers, four priests at a loss. Our teacher said, "You fellows want to know what I thought last week, when those two punks shot that gas station attendant?"

We wanted to know.

"I thought that they ought to hang those g-- d----- punks from the highest tree they could find." Did we understand that? We understood it. "Well, why didn't you preach about that?"

"That won't do."

"Why not?"

"That'd let the genie out of the bottle."

"And you're afraid you'd never get it back in, eh?"

"Right."

"You're saying, 'I can show the darkness, but I'm afraid that if I shine the light of the Gospel on it, nothing will happen.' "

"Exactly."

"You're afraid that belief can't win out over unbelief, is that it?"

"I think so, yes."

"And so you decided not to talk about anything at all."

"I don't understand."

"Belief is about unbelief, isn't it?"

"I understand."

And I began to understand a bit why I really hadn't thought the sermon was so good. The young priest had the pluck, the courage, to look into his own soul and to reveal to us and to himself the rumblings he found there. But of course you've got to have a lot of faith in the house before you can dare admit so much unfaith.

Doubt

In the golden days of radio, the Dutch comedian Wim Kan once did a parody of a morning radio show, including the early morning devotions. After peddling his serious nonsense for a while, he suddenly burst out laughing. When he'd finished, he said, "Hah, if that preacher suddenly burst out laughing, at least you'd know that a real human being was at the other end of the line."

For years I've found that a good joke. A real human being can look at himself and make fun of his own importance; he can tolerate the thought that he isn't God; he knows that his belief and unbelief are quite close to each other, and he keeps in touch with both of them. He doesn't have to impress people with his faith, doesn't have to flirt with his doubts or bury them under a mask of piety.

I've mentioned a television sign-off that I did on the subject "The Lord Is My Shepherd," and how people were interested by my admission that maybe the wish is father to the thought and that the Lord is *not* our shepherd. A "confession of unfaith," so to speak, but many people were hooked by it; it had done them good, somehow had given them room to listen to the confession of faith that came next.

A few days after I'd written that piece, I received from a patient in our hospital a booklet to have a look at. It was called "The Lord Is My Shepherd," and it was published by a society for the spread of the Holy Scriptures. It was subtitled "Comfort for the Sick." There are lovely prayers in that booklet, lovely songs, nice Bible readings. No doubt it's good that there are such books, but I can honestly say that they could be a whole lot better. For in those booklets temptation and doubt are kept hidden out of sight. They do open the door to doubt the tiniest bit, but then it's clear that they themselves are so horrified at what they have done that they immediately slam that door closed with a firm proof text.

Many people in hospitals struggle, like Job among the ashes, with great, anxious questions; but the booklet, it seems, knows nothing of Job and shoots past the bitter questions from the dungheap right to the answers. Psalm 23 is in the booklet, but Psalm 22, the psalm that expresses the feeling of God's abandonment, is nowhere to be found. But Jesus recognized himself in Psalm 22 at his most awful moments; he offered that lamentation up as his prayer. "My God, my God, why have you forsaken me?" That was his prayer of faith as he approached his death. But in this booklet, a suffering person is swept along with a giant pastoral broom to Psalm 23. Those can become empty words, thrown to you from a distance like people feeding pigeons in the park, people who don't want to share your "valley of the shadow of death." All they're interested in is seeing you calm and pious in the green pastures.

Such a booklet gives new credence to the old misconception that temptation and doubt have to be *overcome* in the life of a Christian. But there's an old story from World War II about the R.A.F. pilot who prayed, "O Lord, (if there is a Lord), save my soul (if I have one)." And that story has been around so long that anyone can guess that people find in this doubt of God and self a certain kind of joy.

The growth of our religious life wouldn't be possible without such doubt. Doubt is the forerunner of all growth, says the psychiatrist Ph. Rümke, and therefore doubt should not be laden with guilt but must have a chance to develop. We must neither repress doubt nor glorify it.

In our hospital you often find the finest faith among those who find it hard to believe. Similar ideas are to be found in the writings of Heije Faber and J. H. Van den Berg. Faber has said that the true believer is the person who dares to entertain unbelief as well as belief and that—as he sees it—there is more faith present in some of the expressions of those who resist God than in the words and books of those who seem to be as at home in the Lord's house as if they themselves were the lords of the place. Van den Berg says that he has seen more about God in the writings of various existential philosophers who could only talk about an absent God than in many books about dogmatics.

I remember that just before I left my little parish in the flatlands of North Holland, I was asked to let the congregation hear once again the words of the journalist Van Randwijk. "Is it really so?" wonders Van Randwijk, meditating about the coming of God in Christ. And then he says, "Even if it isn't true, the thought that it is true is so incomparably marvelous that I am prepared to prick up my ears from now until the moment of my death, listening for that news."

Polarization

"My experiences with the conservative and progressive wings of our church," said the bishop's right-hand man, "have taught me that the right wing is not willing to have a dialogue (for dialogue is useless; Rome must speak and then the matter is settled) and that the left wing always talks about a dialogue, but is unable to carry one on."

Snickers among the listeners, because the right heard something ugly about the left, the left heard the right being teased, and those who had suffered in the middle saw both sides "get theirs" and received double joy.

Someone asked how it comes about that left and right understand each other so poorly. This person said that he was weighed down by it in his congregation, and he hoped the bishop's right-hand man could "make a fist," because he himself felt powerless. But that was how the bishop's right-hand man felt, too.

"I'm not a psychologist," he said, and searched the faces in the circle, but everybody there was a theologian, so the group, with bland faces, quickly changed the subject.

★ ★ ★

Partly, I think as penance for my own share in that sinful silence, I promised myself that I'd react to that statement, though a bit late.

"I'm not a psychologist," said the theologian. Well, I've learned to be wary of psychologists who say "I'm not a theologian," because usually what they mean is, "I don't know much about people's dealings with God, and I'd just as soon keep it that way." I suspect that the bishop's right-hand man was really saying a similar thing about the dealings of human beings with one another, and that's rather dangerous, unless the bishop himself sees to it that his *left*-hand man is a psychologist, and that each hand knows what the other is doing: but enough of that.

Up on a Swiss alp, instead of the usual detective novels you're supposed to read on a skiing vacation, I was passing the time piously with a book almost as tension-producing: a doctoral dissertation from Nijmegen University by F. Zonnenberg entitled "Polarization Among Religious." It was a story full of insinuations and violence, set in a monastery, with flawless sleuthing about who-slaughtered-whom, and a great surprise ending.

Members of a monastic community had gotten trapped in polarization; life became unbearable, for it is terrible if brethren cannot dwell together in unity anymore. With their last scrap of faith they'd called for help from outside; yes, they still had enough faith on hand that they dared to call in skilled help. Two psychologists familiar with the situation undertook an investigation.

★　★　★

"Behold how we no longer love each other!" the monks seemed to be saying. "Who are we? What are we really doing to each other? Can things be any different?"

The investigators began their work with an attitude test. For there are rigid people and flexible people, tolerant and intolerant ones, people who find it marvelous if others are different, and people who really can only attack and defend. It appeared that the largest group in this monastery—56 percent—were of a particular personality type: rigid, intolerant, and inclined to find fault with others. But thus far we're only dealing with psychological similarity, for as far as the right is from the left, so far were two attitudes separated in this group: 34 percent rigidly conservative and 22 percent rigidly progressive. This result, by the way, might well indicate that the statement made by the bishop's right-hand man could be corrected a bit, and that neither left *nor* right is capable of having a dialogue. One shouldn't take that as a condemnation. We're dealing here with ultimate values from which a person draws security; they give you a handhold in this dangerous life, so shock and resistance are natural reactions when someone begins to bring down the very roof over your head.

★　★　★

Well, we could say a lot more interesting things about the diagnosis, but I still need to say something about the beginning of the cure.

Shocked by what had been shown to them in the mirror, the monks decided to work on their mutual relationships and to deal with the apparent polarization. They recognized their anxiety about conflict and their powerlessness to deal with it constructively, so they began by practicing listening to one another. But how difficult that seemed after all those years of confusing debate with dialogue, and power grabbing instead of freely looking for truth. Gradually they began to realize how irreverently they'd been jerking around with each other's feelings, and they experienced the renewing power of that old saying by the apostle—that love drives out all fear.

Boxing

The warlike pagans who occupied Holland before Caesar moved north were called Batavians. Well, the Batavian in me likes to watch boxing. Sometimes we get up in the early morning hours just to see how men on the other side of the world try to send each other *out* of the world. I try to put my conscience, which is also wide awake, back to sleep quickly with the rationalization that those brainless men over yonder can't possibly damage each other's brains, just shake them up at the most.

I root for the guy who's winning; I don't like being on the side taking all the blows. Meanwhile, something similar is happening with the loser; as soon as it dawns on him that he can't escape the beating he's taking, he immediately gets close to the guy who's beating him, embraces him, and renders him harmless. "Break it up!" calls the referee, in the name of all "Batavians" who take pleasure in the pain of others and who want to see the mauling begin again. But within a few seconds we see the victim throw himself once again into the arms of his executioner, because it's the only way he's going to escape more pain and humiliation.

★ ★ ★

Well, that's a good illustration of what in learned language we call "identification with the aggressor." In all probability the story of Patty Hearst is a good example. In the middle of the night she was violently kidnaped, and after a few weeks she embraced her kidnaper, and the man's theories, as well. After all this brutality, he told her where to get rid of her not inconsiderable aggression; with coarse words not repeated here her father and her mother and her fiancé were chewed out.

> So long, ma, so long, pa,
> I'm off to the races, ha! ha! ha!

I'm never coming back; I'm ready to die for my new beliefs. Poor kid, it was her only chance to survive.

In Beilen, when a group of Moluccans trying to force the Dutch government to accede to some of their demands hijacked a whole train, we saw the same thing. Those train passengers could have been gunned down at any moment of the day or night. How to survive? Not by doing what you'd like to do: smash the hijackers' faces and curse their theories. It's better to do just the opposite: pat the hijackers on the head, be sympathetic with them, agree with them. "But they were such sincere young men," said a minister on the train. "They read from the Bible every day."

Yes, but the moment they stopped reading, they could easily start shooting; those two things could very well be reconciled with each other. The fact that the Scriptures don't talk about a promised land of Molucca and honey is under the circumstances a life-endangering theology, so just let that alone. "God is good; God heard our prayers," said one of the hostages after everything was over. I just hoped that the widows of the people who were murdered didn't hear *that* gospel.

★   ★   ★

Well, I've been thinking a lot about all that for several weeks now, and I think you can call that "identification with the aggressor," too. You come to a place where you seem to have been abandoned by God, but you can't do what you'd like to do, which is to be "faithless," perhaps to scream at God with coarse words and say, "My God, my God, why have you forsaken me?" No, you say, "God is good, and I'll not want." Sometimes it strikes an honest note if people confess God's goodness. And sometimes it sounds like a TV evangelist, and I don't believe a word of it.

★   ★   ★

"She's in Room 17," said the head nurse, "and she's asked for you a couple of times. She's still a young woman, but . . . well, you'll see."

A young woman, frightened, unsure of herself; you could see it in her face, and you could hear it in the tale of sickness and abandonment she told. "But God helps me so terribly much," she said. "Really!" she added, when she sensed my hesitation. I really didn't know what to say and took a moment to think.

"Say what you think," she said.

"I think you're putting me on," I said.

"No, no, really, if I didn't have God . . ."

"You don't have God," I said, more Batavian than pastoral. And just as I began to get myself back under control, she spoke again, stuffing under her pillow the Bible that a second earlier she'd been waving at me ostentatiously: "I don't pray anymore. God said to me, 'I'm not going to listen to *you* any longer.' God said to me, 'I'm going to teach you a lesson.' That's why I'm here."

"You're God-sick."

"Yes," she said.

A militant woman.

Praying for the Neighbor

There is just a handful of Protestants living in our little village on the river. The Neighbor was one of them. She just died. We are all very close to one another, very involved with one another in our little neighborhood, the folks who live on this side of the village in the bend of the dike. On weddings and anniversaries we make triumphal arches for one another, and when we have funerals we collect money for a nice wreath.

A couple of days after I came to the parish I paid my first call on The Neighbor. She'd found six priests sitting in a row (and the front row, at that!) at my installation a bit too much. She didn't care much for anything ecumenical. She told me how she'd become a widow at a young age, and how her husband, who'd become Protestant to please her, had on his deathbed been received back into the bosom of Holy Mother Church at the instigation of the starch-bosomed nuns in the hospital, and how he'd been buried in the Roman Catholic cemetery. She didn't know exactly where because she'd never been there.

She didn't live far from the Catholic church in those days. A few weeks after her husband's death, she encountered the priest near the church as she was taking her youngest daughter to be baptized. She couldn't help calling out to him, "Y'got the old man, but ya won't get the youngest!" The youngest daughter told me that story herself, and also told me the "delicate" little rhyme that she'd been teased with as a child:

> Protestants are great big monkeys,
> They make noises like the donkeys.
> They won't believe in any God,
> But only in the chamber pot.

She couldn't remember a comparable Protestant fight song.

At The Neighbor's funeral the church was full. Of course, our whole neighborhood was there, but there were also a lot of Catholics; you could tell by the speed at which they took the Lord's Prayer and by the weak singing. Next time I'll have the *De Profundis*, which the Catholic priest abolished in an unguarded moment, in the service. It was a lovely service. We confessed our guilt for the grief our churches had given each other over the years. We prayed for unity and for the ability to honor each other's spirituality, and after that we buried her in the small Reformed cemetery about two miles from her husband. The neighbors provided a lovely floral piece.

The next week some of the Catholics came to tell me that there was some money left over. "Could Mr. Minister say a Mass—or whatever you folks call it?" and then everyone could once again pray for The Neighbor. It would be so appropriate, they said, since next Sunday would have been her birthday. And of course that was a nice coincidence since the Reformed Church—as they all knew—was closed on weekdays. And if Mr. Minister didn't want the money, then they'd buy flowers to put on the "altar," which they could take to the cemetery after the service in a nice little procession. The funeral service had been "such a lovely ceremony"; we'd sung so nicely together, and it was really a pity that The Neighbor herself couldn't have been there.

★ ★ ★

I find it a moving request, and I can hardly tolerate the fact that it worries me. And it embarrasses me, just as it did the other day when I asked the children in the church service what we should pray for. "For my grandfather," said a little girl.

"That's good," I said. "Why do you want to do that?"

"He's dead."

In the prayer I said that sometimes we are sad when we think of grandfather who is no longer with us, and extra sad for grandmother, since she must be thinking about grandfather even more than we do. But that wasn't what that little girl had asked for. She wanted me to do something for her grandfather. But I did something for *her* and for her grandmother, and that's another thing altogether.

"My little girl goes to a Catholic school," her father told me after the service, excusing her and clarifying the situation. "That's what they teach them there."

And are they teaching them something weird? I was always taught that you can't pray for the dead; you can't care for them anymore; they are now in God's care. But I think that Catholics pray for their dead not because they haven't entrusted them to God (and also not because of Purgatory, for that's only smoldering now), but because they trust that God hears their prayers gladly, both for the living and for the dead, and because it is good in God's sight when people plead for each other and do not forget one another's names either in life or in death, or thereafter. And my hunch is that it is pleasing to God if we do indeed plead with him for one another, and ask him not to forget the names of those who have died.

I have no idea how it stands now with The Neighbor and her husband; I'd just as soon not deal with that, but I am really beginning to believe that the Lord will like it if he hears us pray for The Neighbor from time to time when it is her birthday—both Protestants and Catholics, the old and the young, the whole neighborhood. And we ourselves shall like it, too, that's obvious.

Blessing

(1)

A dangerous psychopath: that's what the diagnosis said. So he was shut up in an institution. A tall, gawky fool who for twenty years had been booted around like a football from mother to aunt to a children's home to grandma to foster care to a children's home to a detention center to a prison to a boarding house. Just reading his file takes your breath away. He has a grave crime on his conscience, but he doesn't want to talk about it; he's afraid I'd find him "naughty" rather than "nice," and he'd like to avoid that. At night it's hard for him to get to sleep; he's afraid of the dark, and it's been agreed that if the night nurses ever find him asleep, they'll just put out the light. He is then always found in such circumstances with a rosary in his hands. The nurse comes to tell me to advise the patient for his own peace—both temporal and eternal—to give up that magic ritual and grow up.

What's going on here? In our pathological anxiety to do away with magic, we take away from a poor wretch the only "handhold" he's still got. In our unbelief we teach him that his faith in Mary, who prays "for us sinners now and at the hour of our death," is junk for the kiddies' playroom. And the kid starts living out in the cold, since we give him nothing to take its place.

I asked the nurse if he'd ever considered tucking the guy in like a father or a mother, if he'd ever offered to say a prayer with him, if he ever followed the old Catholic custom and made the sign of the cross on his forehead and used the old prayer of blessing, "Praised be our Lord Jesus Christ."

The nurse asked if I was crazy.

Crazy? So I am. For I don't do any of that, either.

★   ★   ★

I have vivid memories of a brief discussion with the American psychologist Paul W. Pruyser, after we had been analyzing a conversation with a guilt-ridden woman.

"Did you give her your blessing?"

"No."
"Why not?"
"I didn't think of it."
"Why not?"
"I never think of that."

★   ★   ★

"Don't touch," we teach our children, but we ourselves break the habit only with difficulty. It's true for me, at any rate. Last week in a museum in The Hague, I caught the devil from a museum guard who saw me touching an Indian canoe in an exhibition from the American West. But looking wasn't enough for me. I wanted to get closer to that lovely canoe and to the hand of its maker. I get that feeling all over again when I read the Resurrection stories about Mary Magdalene and doubting Thomas; they wanted to touch Jesus; they couldn't believe their eyes but they *could* believe their hands.

We don't lay hands on each other anymore; that language is hardly spoken any longer. Now that I think of it, it's striking to realize with what shriveled-up gestures the blessing, the benediction, is "spoken," instead of being generously given with outstretched arms, the safe wings of mother eagle. In that crabbed gesture I detect a real doubt whether God has the whole world in his hands, or has our names engraved on the palm of his hand. I recognize that doubt, and I know that in it lies one of the sources of my own hesitation to spread my own wings. But then I'm withholding something from people. It's like something withheld from me when a pastor, supposedly giving a benediction, says, "The Grace of our Lord Jesus Christ, and the love of God, and the fellowship of the Holy Spirit with you all."

That's no proper use of language. What is that man saying to me? He's saying, "I stand midway between '*is* with you' and '*be* with you' because I've got a theological and linguistic problem." That's information, but it isn't a benediction. The congregation button up their coats; nobody seems to notice that something special is happening; and, indeed, nothing special *is*.

★　★　★

I'll always remember a Pentecost service at a black church in Kansas City. Not a word about the Holy Spirit, but the Spirit doesn't have to be named in order to get you into its grip. The minister preached about the woman who touched the hem of Jesus' garment. Before the benediction he said, "Now I am going to touch you. And you must touch each other. Please touch. Give each other your hands. Then I'll give you the benediction. God says, 'I love you.' And you need to say to your neighbors on the left and on the right, 'I love you.' "

I was moved. Touched. I lack the simplicity and confidence to say to the farm folk in my village the lines of the children's hymn: " 'Children of one Father, reach out your hands to each other.' Let us celebrate our community tangibly, palpably, with God and with each other."

I'm a remote-control pastor. One who reads Guido Gezelle's poetry in the evening:

> But the sign of the cross has remained
> Written deeply within my head.

Are there people who recognize this flaw in me?

(2)

It happened a year or so ago. On Palm Sunday, the Sunday school children had once again made Easter things, and I suggested that right after the benediction they should march into the church to show the congregation the work of their hands. "Why not *before* the benediction?" asked a leader. Muhammad Ali couldn't have delivered a tougher punch.

The incident flashed into my mind when, in the many letters that I got in reaction to my tale about blessing and laying on of hands, I read one from a doctor in the Dutch Indies, who because of a super-busy practice was often denied the opportunity to go to church, but who, if he had the opportunity, tried to be present at least by the time the benediction was given. *Too bad, he's late again,* the preacher may have thought, but the doctor was happy that he was so wonderfully on time!

In fact I sat breathlessly reading those letters, weeping with those who were weeping over the poverty of contact in pastoral and religious work, happy with the happy about the rare, beautiful moments in life when someone touches you on God's behalf and speaks words that win your heart. But we are no longer trained for that; we have buried our talents. "We must learn once more to believe with our whole bodies: dreaming, sitting quietly, laying on hands, caressing, and kissing," writes Willem Berger in *Liturgy by the Sickbed*. And as long as we haven't learned that, Sunday school teachers will give us a whack on the knuckles and send us back to the dunce's corner at seminary. And you won't learn it there, either.

The Bible is full of preaching in sign language, and mothers bring their children to Jesus "so that he could touch them and lay hands upon them." Those are gripping tales, but we make lovely sermons out of them, expensive syrups from the drug store instead of mother's milk, as Luther expressed it. Meanwhile many people suffer from a taboo on intimacy. For example, when a new preacher is ordained, you often see the ordaining pastors and elders in a ring making a kind of sagging Hitler salute over the unsuspecting, kneeling ordinand's head, or else they're playing slap hands. It'd be better if we were to give the new minister a secular sort of clap on the shoulders, like dubbing a knight, as a charge to him to conduct himself like a knight.

Now I'd like to come back to the denial of the verb in the blessing: The grace of our Lord Jesus Christ, and the love of God, and the fellowship of the Holy Spirit with you all. I heard that lame text again recently. The preacher had offered evidence in his sermon that he knew God well and himself poorly. And so we had no contact with each other, and in that case the benediction hangs there in midair and isn't even a blessing in disguise, for there is nothing there to seal; so in this case it was a double failure.

"Be with you" I find rather a weakening of the promise, but it's certainly possible, I think, that some people consider "is with you" too strong and too presumptuous on their lips. With such people I can certainly pray the benediction. But personally I say, though it's sometimes contrary to experience, "The Lord *is* my shepherd"; and I say to others, as well, "The Lord *is* your shepherd." I find, moreover, that the other person has to say "Amen" to that blessing. He himself has to say yes and amen to it; the one who blesses, blesses, and the one who is blessed lets it be known that he knows he is in God's hand and accepts that God has laid hold of him. "Be it done to me according to your word," says the Virgin Mary. She was not raped, the theologian Van Ruler teaches us, and let those who really want to receive the blessing quickly say amen to it.

★　★　★

Catholic children once received from their fathers or mothers, before going to sleep, the sign of the cross on their foreheads. "Praised be Jesus Christ," the parent would say, and on hearing that the child would answer, "For ever and ever. Amen."

That a mystery should be pictured and mediated physically speaks of a primitiveness that we have behind us but hopefully also before us. Guido Gezelle remembers with gratitude that "the sign of the cross has remained written deeply within my head," and many letter writers remember gratefully how, at special moments in their lives, they were allowed to experience God's nearness in words and symbols, and knew themselves or another (someone alive or dead) to be blessed.

"Did your mother once do that, too, make the sign of the cross on your forehead?" I asked a Catholic man in our village, a genuine "river rat" from the banks of the Maas. He gave me a sidelong glance, but when he saw that I intended the question seriously, he said, very adult and very childlike, "Sometimes she still does."

Something

"I believe that there *is* something."

The man looked outside, slantingly upward.

"I really do believe there's something."

It has struck me that people often look outside when they are saying that. Out the hospital window, through the prison bars, at home: human eyes hunt for space, for light, for the skies when they are asking you not to number them among those who believe that there's nothing.

Yes, they may seldom or never come to church and may know little or nothing of the Bible. They'll probably have more questions than answers without even being any too aware of that—just as long as you don't think that, spiritually, they live in a flatland. For they really believe that life has still another dimension than just concern for your daily bread and some diversion at appropriate moments—look, the world didn't just come into existence all by itself. It must have a purpose, a meaning, and, although I don't know what, there is *something*. The world isn't a closed system; there's an origin, a purpose, and a meaning. And although I don't know much about it, there *is* an opening.

And their eyes seek an opening in the closed room and look out, slantingly upward.

★   ★   ★

Let me admit honestly that I've learned only slowly to listen with respect to that faith statement of people that there is "something." In my pride I thought that belief only a scanty one. "Does that 'something' *say* anything?" I asked, uncharitably taking aim at their poverty instead of beginning to rejoice with them at their riches.

People who confide to you that there must be something are looking for a closer relationship. They don't want to belong to those who think that they themselves are all there is and don't bother with origin and meaning and purpose as long as soup's on the fire. Living like that would be suffocating for them, a stifling place where they couldn't draw a breath—and their eyes are looking for the space they keep telling you about. You're supposed to be able to sympathize with that; you know what they're talking about, don't you? After all, you are that man who represents that spaciousness, that light, that mighty wind from heaven, aren't you?

Often enough people will add that you may certainly call that "something" God, if you don't mind the fact that they just stop at that.

"Great faith" is too great for them, too unapproachable; they are just ordinary people, and they just believe ordinary things. "Small faith"—*that* they can be more concrete about, because it is more concrete. They tell you what mother always said, and that they contribute to the church, and that they are always silent for a moment before meals. They can show you a Bible with a history and can tell you what they felt when they happened to go into that church last summer. It often seems that those who could only be vague in "great faith" dare to have strong feelings about its shrinkage and dare to entrust themselves to those feelings.

★ ★ ★

In Brabant I know people who find it very difficult to pray. Once in a while they bicycle to the chapel of the Little Brother of Megen. A good man: that's what you see in the image of this Franciscan monk carved on his gravestone in a little chapel of the Franciscan monastery. The Little Brother of Megen always lived close to God and close to people; now he is with God. Anyone who finds it difficult to pray to God can take his bicycle and make a pilgrimage to the Little Brother, burn a candle there, and leave a note in the stone folds of his robe. In the dialect of East Brabant, ordinary people write about their grief and their hard lives, and sometimes about their gratitude. Our Little Brother will surely be able to explain to God why we don't pray to him directly. He can translate our Brabant speech just right, and he knows when you shouldn't bother our Lord. And he knows what kind of creatures we are.

Body and Soul

The town lies just a bit off to the side of the highway south of Dijon, in the middle of Burgundy. If you take a trip to France, you should leave the streams of vacation traffic behind and breathe in the quietness of this little wine-making town.

Right in the heart of the town there's a building out of the Middle Ages—built, to be precise, in 1442 by Nicolas Rolin, chancellor of Philip the Good, Duke of Burgundy. With a little luck, you'll see the sun reflected off the glazed roof tiles; you can also tell that they were installed with love. In fact, care and love are worked into the whole place, including the interior, which was what we'd come to see.

"The great room of the poor"—236 feet long, 46 feet across, and 52 feet high—looks like a church. But it's no church. It's a sickroom. On either side we see "cupboard beds" surrounded with red cloth, in which the sick lay, alone, or, when things were badly crowded, in twos. If you were about to die you were kept separate, not for the weird reasons that *we* usually have, but so that you would be warm; the isolation area was near the kitchen behind the stoves.

At Rolin's expense you would be gently cared for by valiant nuns with great winged caps; it was hard to tell whether they'd just landed or were about to take off for heaven. From your bed you could see the altar, and you could follow the Mass. And afterward the priest came around with the sacraments. The nuns sang in the choir.

★　★　★

What could the nuns do? Not much, medically speaking. Nurse you. Bleed you. Purge you. Make medicine from their own herb garden. More than that? Sing. Pray. The guide who led us around took on a compassionate tone of voice when he was telling us about the primitive conditions of those days, and at such moments, of course, you become aware all over again of the gigantic leaps of modern medicine. And yet. The five centuries between then and now have not only brought gains.

The guide talked about how one was admitted to the hospital. One of the nuns of our Lord's flying brigade stood in the hall waiting for you and immediately took you to the confessional, he said. Mumbling in the ranks of the tourists. "Think about it a moment. It's good that we don't do it that much anymore. Imagine—you came to the door sick unto death, and you had to confess your sins first!"

Then you were put to bed, but you were cleverly manipulated again, because, whether you wanted to or not, you had to look at the altar. And behind it a large painting, attributed to Rogier Van der Weyden, a sermon in pictures. It showed—well, what do you think the painter would put on display for the sick folk in God's hospital?

★　★　★

Don't be shocked. A portrayal of the Last Judgment. The end of time is there; the trumpets are sounding; the earth shakes; the graves are opening; you see the dead rising; and now they step before the judgment seat. The Archangel Michael tries to handle the scales as carefully as possible, and Mary sits alongside. "Mother Mary, pray for us sinners, now and at the hour of our death and in the hour of the Last Judgment." Mary is there, and she is praying for us sinners. Some are ascending to heaven. Up above, God himself stands waiting for them in a brilliant light. Some are descending into hell. Hmmm, I've said that rather too nicely; for it's gruesome what is happening there. Devils with tridents are torturing the damned in pools of fire, and, wailing, the damned disappear in the depths.

And that's what you looked at the whole blessed day, in that hotel of God! Twentieth-century visitors shake their heads, give the guide a franc, and race on to the beaches where, every day, God maketh his sun to shine on the just and the unjust. What one might wish at that point is that people would be able to look at that painting more openly, more receptively, more freely. I am personally more struck by our primitiveness than by that of medieval society! Sure, I can say a lot of unpleasant things about confession, too. How the church has used it manipulatively, how it was more and more emptied out until its real meaning was no longer there at all. And I know how, right up to the present moment, obedience and faithfulness to the group have been forced, and authentic faith crippled, by the fear of hell and damnation. And I know, as well, that it was altogether too easy and too simple to make direct connections between sin and sickness.

★　★　★

But having said all that, I want to say this, too. In our own day, we know that often, oftener than we think, there's a connection between a person's life and that person's sickness. But with that knowledge we do little that's useful. The nuns in the Hotel of God had just a bare understanding of that. But they did something with that understanding. What, after all, does that confessional bench mean, what does that holy picture story on the wall mean, if not an invitation to a sick person to take his life in his hands, to put the good and evil in his life before the face of God? What is it but a question of whether your way of life leads to health or illness, whether your illness is merely destiny or something you've brought upon yourself?

In our own day we play Mr. and Mrs. Clever about the unity of body and soul. In the meantime we pull that unity apart. But in the Hôtel Dieu at Beaune you see the inseparable unity in this sickroom that's a church, this church that's a sickroom. God's guests we are. And we are kindly but firmly asked to think about what that might mean. Illness asks for contemplation about meaning and gives an opportunity for it, just as a vacation gives you a chance to look at your life from a distance, as it were from above, looking at it with God.

★　★　★

Those nuns knew little or nothing about sickness. But I know for sure that they saved the lives of many people.

They committed their folks to God, or in French, *à Dieu*.

Do-It-Yourselfer

"I guess it's OK for you to sit with me,"said the man in the plaster cast. "But I don't have anything more to do with faith."

"I'm a specialist in that," I said.

Why so aggressive?

The man lay there dealing with being sick the same way he was used to handling good health: full of bombast and chatter. He filled your ears with rot about his wonderful car which was now totaled, about the expected decline of his business, about the "cute little nursies" with whom you could have fun, about the doctors, hard workers who earned every penny they had. He kept words flipping in the air like a juggler, and deftly avoided talking about anything real.

He'd made it, he thought. And from scratch. First, a booth in the market—but his feet got too cold standing outside. Bought a business in Arnhem—a cigar store, poor business. He switched over to do-it-yourself stuff. A regular gold mine. He didn't want the profits to line the purses of those tax collectors, so he opened a second store. It went like a house afire. Opened another store, this time in Apeldoorn. A deluxe life, that's what he had now. Except for that accident.

★　★　★

A couple of days later I saw him again. The storm was clearly over; now he was quiet. He showed me a child's drawing. Flowers. "For Papa, from Simone, age 9." I saw that the man quickly wiped away a few tears. I asked him if he could summon the courage to cry for real. He could. And he told about Simone. She'd spent three-quarters of an hour with him. Completely alone. Such a chatterbox! He hadn't known she could talk like that. And so smart!

"I must be crazy," he said. "I never see that kid. There's no time. I'm working myself to death. In the summer I say to my wife, 'Here's some money, take a plane and go to Spain with the kids.' And they go. I can't get away. I only went with them once. And then I was on the phone more than I was on the beach. My wife said that she'd just as soon I wasn't along. She often says it's just crazy to work like that. But what am I gonna do?

"Simone can really draw well, don't you think? Nine years old. Another nine years and she'll be eighteen. And then she'll leave home. And I'll have had no daughter, and she won't have had a father. And another year or so, and the old heart will refuse to keep going. Into the hospital again. And maybe I won't come out that time. Instead, I'll see Saint Peter. Y'know what he'll say? 'Who's this?' I'll say, 'Ter Horst.' 'I don't know you,' says Peter. 'Ter Horst, from Arnhem,' I say. 'Really, I don't recognize the name,' says he. 'What have you done in your life?' 'Me?' I say. 'I'm the ter Horst with all the do-it-yourself stores.' 'And what else?' asks Peter. 'Nothing else,' I have to answer."

★ ★ ★

Still another time he's reading. Short stories. "Are they any good?" I ask.

"Doesn't do a thing for me," he says. "It's all about nothing at all. He just barfs up words. He thinks he's a great gift to the world. But he's just a shot of bitter medicine. Look here, see what he writes at the end of this story: 'Amsterdam, October 19, 1975.' As if he's created I don't know what. 'On this day in Amsterdam I gave the world the gift of this story.' But the man has nothing to say. And he never will. He's never experienced a crisis like the one I'm in now. He . . ."

He goes on scolding. *But why's he so angry?* I ask myself. *Is he angry with himself?* And I said, "It's a story without any depth, isn't it? It's all about life on the surface, 'full of sound and fury, signifying nothing.' You're disgusted by that. It looks like a temptation for you, a temptation that you'd like to drive away with all your might."

★ ★ ★

Later still I met him on a park bench. He'd just gone for a walk in the woods. "My God, it's beautiful in there," he said. "That Boss of yours really knows how to arrange things. I sat there looking at just one tree for the longest time. That tree was there long before I came along. And it'll be there long after I'm gone. And that tree's beginning to come alive again. Everywhere you look that mighty thing is coming into bloom again. It's just beautiful, just beautiful."

His story moved me. How that man himself had begun to bloom again! Racing along year after year through that wooded part of Holland between Arnhem and Apeldoorn, never seeing a tree, busy beating the rest of the world. Then through Simone's lilies of the field and one tree of the Lord's he discovers that he's gained the whole world and lost his soul. "Listen, just tell your Boss . . ."

"Why don't you tell him yourself?" I asked.

He wondered if some Sunday afternoon he might walk in these woods again.

"On the sabbath," I said. "With Simone. And the other kids. And your wife. You'd really like to share all this with them, wouldn't you?"

"Yeah," he said. "I hope I'll be able to do that. I hope so."

And after a moment: "It's time I stopped acting as if I weren't there."

Punishment

Justice, the lady who wears a blindfold while she's weighing things and people in her scales so that she can operate without regard to persons, has always had little power to attract me. I think she should use her eyes and carefully decide whether punishment serves any useful purpose. For years I've been announcing provocatively both inside and outside prison walls that I strongly believe in "class justice," and of course it's all the same to me whether someone is set in high places or is one of the schlemiels, the poor suckers.

Distributions of justice that are exactly alike are an absurdity; there are no two people exactly alike. One of the newspapers, I notice, thinks differently, and labeled the session of Parliament aimed at dealing with Prince Bernhard and the Lockheed affair a "church service." If they meant by that that the whole thing was rather wearisome and that very little was said that was sparkling or original, I'd have to bow my head humbly; that's how it does go all too often in the church—mine, too.

But if they mean that kindness and compassion left their mark on this meeting, the comparison is pleasant, indeed. I followed the entire session from inside a prison. That makes you even more sensitive to what's really going on. I was sitting next to a chauffeur who, in spite of the fact that he'd been drunk behind the wheel, had been allowed to keep his driver's license on the grounds that they didn't want to punish him twice by taking away his job, a particularly charming form of class justice. That man had an especially keen understanding that those Members of Parliament in The Hague judging the prince were aware of who it was they were dealing with. All except the incomprehensible, inexorable pacifists. These peacemakers are not blessed; they want to see blood flow.

★   ★   ★

We were happy with the plan of Bas De Gaay Fortman, one of the members of Parliament, to weigh the value or lack of value of punishment in all cases with the same care as was used in this case. That is a lot better than the "lock them up and no more nonsense" that a (sad to say) prominent politician uses from time to time when he's pretending to be the "voice of the people."

For that matter, my first reaction is to say that that's exactly what I think. For in the depths of my mind I'm also a tabloid reader. Tabloids are newspapers after my own heart, because my heart is evil and guilty. After that, when I have the feeling that people have space to listen just a little bit, I say that I know how to repent if I can get in touch with my knowledge and my experience (after that first emotional outburst which has been nurtured on anxiety). And I become my old self completely again when I've been walking for an hour or so along the cell corridor.

You ought to come with me some evening. We won't gloss over the terrible things for which these people had to be segregated from the rest of society. In fact, maybe we'll talk about them in all their gruesome details. It's not hard to loathe the men here. But I also know that it's not hard to love them, either, and you'd understand why.

Surely I'd take you to visit the young man who took his wife's life. He doesn't trust me, and he's right; life's taught him not to trust anybody. He's close to complete loss of hope, and sometimes he seems to allow you to come a little closer to that. He stares at his hands. "Hard to imagine it, eh?" I say. "It was fate," he says. "It just had to be." He sits like Adam in the bushes hiding from God. And what about forgiveness, I wonder, because forgiveness has to do with guilt, and he can't even look into that deep well.

Would a stiff sentence have had any preventive value? We know better than that. Hate blinds people just as love does. Rational considerations have little braking power in stress situations. Society can't have him around for the time being. I understand that; but what's supposed to happen to him here? Can he learn in these surroundings to believe in other people, in himself, in God? I'm just asking.

Karl Barth said that he thought punishment Christian only as a measure of our care, and I have to think about that often. I don't simply advocate tolerance. I advocate an attitude that can bring healing, growth, reconciliation, and redemption. If *in*tolerance contributed to that, I'd be for it. And now that this piece too is beginning to sound like a "church service," a quotation from Bonhoeffer would be in order: "Whoever despises a man can never be able to have real contact with him. We have to learn to see people less on the basis of their deeds and omissions, and more on the basis of their pain."

Amen.

Jabbok

I'm not sleeping again, and that's really miserable. I'm having bad dreams again. Tomorrow I've got to come see you again. "Well, what did you dream?" you're going to ask me. I get a rotten taste in my mouth just thinking about it.

How many weeks have I been coming to see you? I don't even know why I go each time, and the chance that others will find out I'm coming gets bigger all the time. Don't they ever have problems? Do they solve them all themselves? I'd really like to know. For that matter, I'd really like to know something from you. Do you talk to people about what I tell you? No, I don't think you do—not that you're so trustworthy; I don't believe in trustworthy people—but just because you forget me the minute I walk out the door. Or *do* you think about me? It's your job to look at people, isn't it, to see them floundering and in pain, to see them doubting God and everything and everybody and most of all themselves. You look at all that like a biologist looks at a beetle. But if it's your wife who's depressed, do you do your pastoral trick then?

★　★　★

Forgive me. But it's so wrenchingly difficult to need you. In fact, you're the one person I still trust a little bit. I've told you a lot about myself—thoughts and deeds and longings of which I'm sometimes so terribly ashamed. And you've listened carefully to it all, and you haven't judged me. It's really done me good that you listened and tried to understand it all a little, and the other day I got the joyful feeling that you really do believe in me and that I'm just a little bit worth your time. You said, "A wonderful child of God." For a moment I thought you were making fun of me.

★　★　★

Indeed, I still think so, because you never really make any demands on me. Can I give you something, too, or can I only come and get things from you? Do I have anything to offer you? We have a tidy sharing of roles, and *you* maintain it very carefully: you the helper, I the helpless. Gives you a good feeling, doesn't it? Yes, how come you're so interested in me? Am I one of your interesting cases? Why do you listen to all that human misery, and why are you constantly meddling with everybody?

Come to think of it, you have an awfully squalid job. You go through life as the Great Doer of Good, and by and by you'll go upsy-daisy into heaven, but meanwhile you're walking on our backs, pal. Did you ever think about that? If you just have enough doubters around you, you could get to be the Lord.

You're a strong one, and you collect weaklings, don't you? That's *your* weakness, but you know better than to admit that, because then where would you be with your Messiah complex? Yes, where would you be if all the wretches and bums like us weren't around? A beachcomber without any driftwood. You'd better hope that Jesus on that cloud is going to wait awhile, because when the former things are passed away your kingdom is at an end, pal.

★ ★ ★

You know, I really should be telling you all this tomorrow. But I won't dare. Even if I did, you wouldn't be knocked off your pins. You'll already know what I want to say, even before I've said it. Good heavens, you're a bit like God himself. And really, I admire your strength and your courage, and it's just fine that I can't get at you with all my endless yammering.

I've got a feeling that I wouldn't know how to cope without you, because I need somebody who's big and level-headed, somebody I can trust and who loves me just a little bit. But that's childish. I have to grow up, stand on my own two feet.

But suppose I grew up, knew how to plug the gaps, used all my strength to succeed in shutting off all that self-pity. Suppose it no longer bothered me what people said about me. Suppose I became my true self and still was nobody, nothing, nowhere! I don't dare think about that, for then I'd know for sure what I only suspect now: that it would have been better if I hadn't been born. If I don't change, I'll come to a dead end. And if I do change?

Why should I change? Why don't you take me just as I am? And if you think that change is so necessary, why don't you change me? I mean, what did you do to get where you are? You didn't have to do a lick of work to get there, did you? It's all a matter of grace, to borrow a word from that language of yours. Well, since you know so well just what and where my problem is, why don't you solve it? Why do I have to do everything myself? You know how much you torment me and how afraid I am to take the lid off the well and look down inside. And you sit on the edge while I descend. You know, I don't believe that you really understand what agony is and that you can go just plain crazy from it. You're far too sane, and that's a handicap, did you know that? I bet that I know deeper depths than you do; I've been in places you never even dreamed of. Tell you what: I'm really more human than you! And I wonder if you've ever known real temptation. I think you just get a good kick out of mine.

Do you really want me to grow, to change? If I were you, I'd find it difficult not to be needed anymore. And another thing: if I fail, if I really can't go any farther, then it'll be my fault. You'll never be the cause of it. Unless I get better. Don't you see that you use projection, too?

★ ★ ★

But I use it, too, and more than you. I think I'm terribly unreasonable. No, you don't have to tell me that I'm confused: I know that perfectly well. But I can't change it very well yet. I just hope that you understand me a little, that you have patience with me, and that you won't let me go until you bless me—then maybe I'd be able to stand on my own two feet.

Now I'm going to try to get some sleep.

Do *you* ever lie awake?

Sorry.

Dying

(1)

Caring for the dying is "in" these days. Not long ago I tried to say something about it from a pastoral point of view for a large group of people. I found that creepy. Here was a room full of people looking for a place where death is given some serious consideration, looking for the strength to hang on when they're with dying people and realizing that they're mortal, too.

That last part is especially important, I think, and for that reason I chose to place my emphasis on that, and to talk about holding on and letting go.

★ ★ ★

I told the simple story of a woman who'd worked hard all her life, became sick, and had to let go of one possibility after another. She had to let go of her active, mastering ego, but came to understand that she could hold on to her contemplative, observing ego. She tried to draw up the balance sheet of her life before the Lord, and when she'd finished doing that, very little was left to be said. She waited in silence for God's mercy, and every day I came to wait with her for a little while.

The last time I sat with her, I took her hand and stroked it, and she stroked mine; that was a moving scene. Then came the moment when I had to let go. That was difficult, and I said so; and we wept. I asked her if it was true that when you have to leave each other you're still not out of God's hands. She thought that was so, and so did I. In the doorway I turned around for a moment. She waved her white hand, a little dove. And with my hand I made the sign of the cross; I work in a Catholic hospital, and the habit is catching.

Holding on and *letting go*: the church used to have a lot to say about that. But nowadays the church has less and less to say. That's made room for an open and freer dealing with such things as sexuality. A lovely gain, but an ugly loss comes with it: mortality is suppressed, death is denied. We have come to believe that you only live once, and as long as there's life we can eat, drink, and be merry, and we're not yet grieving about the leaving, because that's a waste of time, and where could we go anyway? Our forebears didn't have to manage time so greedily, because they believed in eternity. We're critical of the way they did that; they sometimes equated heaven with escaping from the responsibilities of earthly life. But in those days *heaven* was not a dirty word, and there was the chance that you could live less covetously, think less egocentrically.

You didn't need to hold on so tightly, because you believed that our Lord wasn't about to let you go.

★ ★ ★

In our village we held an evening service last week. (We don't often do that.) We sang several lovely evening hymns, and I noticed that in all those hymns our forebears worshiped with an awareness of death, exercising the art of dying in the midst of their living. In letting the day pass from their hands—thanking, confessing, complaining, questioning—they paused at the thought of the evening of life awaiting them, when they would have to let *all* their days pass from their hands.

From the psalms we read, "Let our prayer come before you as a fragrant offering, the uplifting of our hands as an evening offering," and we saw before us that man who, worn out from grubbing in the earth, has laid aside his implements, looked up, and lifted up his hands to heaven—empty hands like doves. The day is not snatched away from him; he gives it up out of his hands. That is how he will also want to die, someday. Life will not be taken from him; he will give up his spirit willingly. He hopes to be able to say, "Into your hands I commend my spirit."

The people in my village asked if we couldn't have evening services more often, worshiping in the twilight as the day dies, the horizon narrows, and one's view is turned inward.

★ ★ ★

I want to return to that story of the dying woman. I find that story beautiful but also dangerous, for dying is often anything but beautiful. Experts on dying are very popular. They speak about acceptance and the road to acceptance, but that can get to be some kind of norm, some kind of law. The person who doesn't come to acceptance and the worker who doesn't know how to get a dying person to that kind of heaven are both missing the boat somehow. At least that seems to be the message.

But someone who has lived unfreely, spastically, will often not be able to die in any other way than he has lived: unfreely, spastically. Why not admit that? If you've only learned to conjugate the verb *to have* all your life, you'll find it hard, I think, to conjugate the verb *to be* at the final parting.

A man died who had never accepted his life and who now wasn't accepting his death, either. It was really difficult for the people around him to accept that, but it was their problem and not his. He lay there cursing, and he died as he had lived: under protest.

Elisabeth Kübler-Ross taught me not to get confused about people who in dying shake their fists at heaven. "God can take it," she said. When I think of "letting go," I also try to think of letting go of what in yourself and in others is unfinished, damaged, confused. Old aches and sores. God will make everything new, I believe.

(2)

We were celebrating the last Sunday of the liturgical year—remembering our dead. People went to God with emptiness in their hearts, and there were prayers that God would fill that emptiness. But it's my experience that God doesn't do that. That always used to make me sad, and I thought I was the only one who thought so until I found in Bonhoeffer the consolation that this was his experience, too. From prison he wrote that in his experience God leaves the emptiness empty, so that we should be bound to each other, even if only by our pain. We mustn't try compulsively to fill the emptiness, he says, but try to accept and persevere.

Gratitude, he discovered, changes the pain of remembering into quiet joy. It becomes a gift of great price; from time to time you look at it and grow quiet.

★   ★   ★

Sunday I named in silence the names of those who left an empty place in me this year. One of them I had known for only a few weeks: a simple man of about fifty who, as they say, was "a couple of bricks short of a full load." Shortly after his admission to our hospital, it was evident that all we could do for him was to help him die. Later it looked as if he could do that rather well for himself. With his small vocabulary he could tell about his life very nicely, about its richness, its poverty. He had never married, "because of my speech defect," he said matter-of-factly. He offered us his feelings and his thoughts "unfiltered," and was surprised when he created confusion among us with his simple questions, such as, "Do you think I'll die this week?"

On Sunday afternoons he went driving to take leave of his neighbors, his boss, his acquaintances. For a particular Saturday night he'd gotten permission from the doctor to say good-bye to his friends in his local bar. The daughter of the owner told me later how that had gone.

Late that evening he sat on the bar and called for silence. He told them that he had to go back to the hospital and that he wouldn't be coming to the bar anymore, because he was going to die. He thanked them all for their friendship. And then he called for one last round of drinks on him. The owner filled the glasses. After he'd paid (bar owners are often very good psychologists), he shook hands with everyone and disappeared. His last communion. When he'd left, a couple of the men in the bar began to cry.

Finally he took leave of his family. But death was taking its time, and he didn't want to wait any longer. I got the feeling that he was trying to hurry his end by these good-byes, and I told him that. He said I was right, and that it was stupid of him to put such pressure on the Lord. He talked a lot about heaven, with awe and with expectation. *Out of the mouths of babes*, I thought, and that very moment I heard him say that Jesus had said, "Let the little children come to me," and that he figured that went for him, too.

★　★　★

People can talk about heaven in various ways. Like a child. Or in desperation, as a scream from a horrid existence, like that man in an American prison where I worked who committed suicide, and who'd laid down on his table a little Bible opened to the passage that if our hope is built on Christ only for *this* life, we are the most miserable of all men.

Heaven can also be used by people as a defense against the flood, the horror of destruction. They let the cup of sorrow pass them by, as it were, by means of a premature flight into a belief in eternal life. The priest whom I heard confessing (in the middle of a group of pious types) that he found death horrifying was judged completely out of order and quickly silenced. "Unbelief" wasn't tolerated, and so of course the chance was lost to explore what belief is all about.

★ ★ ★

There are also those who talk of heaven as if they already have a ticket in their pockets. They see themselves as a lovely little gift to God, and they never wonder if the Lord of heaven might think otherwise. They think about the Lord very little, because secretly they think that *they* are the Lord. Erik Erikson has said that the first step toward faith is the acquisition of the knowledge that one is not God, but many keep dreaming that they're the center of the universe and that sun and moon and stars bow before them. They can't imagine that the Lord could ever do without them, and even if they *confess* that they're just a bad odor in God's holy nostrils, they're convinced in their hearts that their lives will be "held over by popular demand" in heaven because here on earth they were so very successful.

Once I sat in on a conversation that my American prison chaplain colleague had with a prisoner who constantly changed the subject to the hereafter because he was scared to death (his feelings were not hard to understand) of the here and now. My colleague thought it best for the immediate and the eternal good of his client to take his toy away from him, and shouted, "My dear man, there is no such place as heaven!"

Later on we evaluated this pastoral/therapeutic maneuver, and started talking about our own expectations of the future. My colleague was a recovering alcoholic, and his struggle against self-indulgence had cost him a great deal. "Do you know when I'll get to heaven?" he asked.

I've had to mull over his answer many times. He said, ". . . When I stop believing in it."

Tolerance

I'll start with a childhood memory.

I attended a Christian school, a "school with the Bible," as we say in Holland, in my case even with the cheerful Bible. We used to begin the new week with devotions, and so we sang happily:

Fresh as the morning, aware of its power,
An eagerness for life streams through my veins.
Eager to lay hand to the plow,
Eager to back weak ones up,
Eager for the world and for the One who created it
And who calls me to my work.

In short, we sat there full of eagerness, and that was even encouraged. On the piano stood Jesus, the way Thorwaldsen saw him, a meek man; he looked like the Jesus in that picture where the great friend of children has surrounded himself with a Chinese girl, a black boy, an Eskimo, and two whites. In other words, I learned tolerance very early, learned to take a broad view. But our tolerance didn't extend (it was wartime) to the little daughter of a member of the Dutch Nazi party. We felt a great eagerness to knock that weak one down, and we did it, too. The teacher said that we had to love her, but we decided that there were limits. I still have bad feelings about that, and I think that's good.

It was a grim time. Educational materials were scarce, and so we had to make do with an ultraconservative Reformed history book. Next to William of Orange the one who took up the most space was Abraham Kuyper [founder of the Free Reformed Church], of all people! The fine points of the Synod of Dordt were also disclosed to us: "The remonstrants taught so-and-so. The counter-remonstrants instead taught such-and-such. The counter-remonstrants were right." And with that triumphant final note the chapter drew to a close. Coaching me, my mother asked, "What did the remonstrants teach?"

I told her.

"And the counter-remonstrants?"

I served that up, too. And then I tossed in as an extra, "And the counter-remonstrants were right." I won't soon forget my mother's perplexity at this presumptuous stupidity. But it confused me.

"Suppose the teacher asks who was right?"

"Then you say that you don't know."

"But then I'll get an *F*!"

★   ★   ★

In America I received an invitation to mediate between a progressive group and a conservative one in a monastery. Each group was sure it was right. Before I went, I consulted Paul Pruyser, the psychologist of religion.

He said, "You must see to it that they talk about their faith. And then you must pay attention to the kind of language they use. They'll talk about their faith as if it were their beloved. They 'cherish' their thinking, they 'hang on to' it as if they were hanging on to mother's skirts, they are 'faithful' to promises once given, their belief is 'dear' to them."

And that makes sense, because they've taken on the faith of beloved people. It is the "faith of their fathers"; it still smells of mother and of teachers they loved. Those are the people they identified with, the people they became a part of. It's a form of loyalty to hold on to truths they held on to and to reject what they always rejected.

The person who learned from his mother that the counter-remonstrants were right keeps to his mother's beliefs, and his own, by rejecting the beliefs of the remonstrants. Many people feel themselves bound to follow the faith of the people to whom they are bound. To give an example, I am bound to the belief that it's always hard to figure out who's right, and that Jesus holds a lot of strange people on his lap.

Surely this is one of the reasons why conversions let loose such deep feelings in parents or children. "It's over between me and my child," says a mother at such a time. And the "fallen-away" child can stand the voices of condemnation within himself only if they are fully balanced by voices of approval in a new, love-filled relationship.

Pruyser thought, rightly and reasonably, that I should take a still broader view; he taught me to listen more attentively to people's faith histories. He unmasked my eagerness to convert people, my missionary zeal, as part of a search for my own security; the more people who believe what I believe, the more likely it is that my faith is right! I caught the vision that people change only when they are in a love-filled relationship. And that my own faith did not so much fall out of the heavens as it was shaped (and misshaped) by the people who taught me to walk and who taught me history; it's conditioned as well by socio-economic factors. And that's true of everybody else's faith, too.

My faith has changed, by the way. There's no Thorwaldsen Jesus on our piano. My faith will change again, perhaps it will even disappear; who knows? I hope people will deal respectfully with the faith I have now.

Some "evangelical" guy asked me recently why I have so much difficulty with evangelical Christianity. That's what I have trouble with. He is claiming the word *evangelical* for himself. I get extremely intolerant with such intolerance.

Ain't I right, teacher?

Cross-Eyed Angels

(1)

Years ago, I read *Cross-eyed Angel*, the story of a father who has a son with Down's syndrome. One image from that story has always stayed with me: the father tells how he constantly but vainly tries to pull the boy into his world, how he measures the boy with his own yardstick. By doing that, the man makes himself unhappy and denies the boy the right to his own world—that is, until the man realizes that he must no longer try to re-create the boy according to his own image and likeness, but must leave him in his world, just as you have to leave a lovely water plant where it is, in that other world of water and algae. Take it into your own world and you've got nothing but a pitiful batch of dregs in your hands; but leave it in its own element, and then it can unfold; it can be lovely and beautiful. So it is with a Down's syndrome child; in his own world he can be beautiful, too, one of God's angels, be it a cross-eyed one.

★ ★ ★

I had to think of that story, that image, again when I read *A House Too Far?*, published to commemorate the twenty-fifth anniversary of Maria Roepaan, an institution for retarded people in Ottersum. Three staff members wrote that book "from the lives of six retarded people." They did it with love, respect, and wisdom. A fourth staff member created lovely photographs to go with the text. Just as with the father of the cross-eyed angel, I was struck by the way they look at these children. You sense in that book the struggle to learn that kind of perception, to teach it to yourself and to one another. One of the stories is about little Mary. In the papers requesting her admission is written, "Mary is an old-looking Mongoloid woman." The first report about her after her admission, written by the administrative staff, starts by saying, "Mary is a jolly fat Mongoloid." The report from the outsiders continues, "What is striking is her enormous sluggishness." The first report from Maria Roepaan says, "She is indeed quite slow, but is perfectly capable of running fast. For example, she has a little satchel, and if you take if from her and run, she'll run after you to get it back."

It all depends on how you look at it. In this connection, another striking story is one about the struggle of a mother to accept her retarded son. "It is as if you were flying a kite. At the beginning it keeps diving at the ground, and you begin to despair. It takes a long time, but now it has found its balance in the clear blue sky."

The fathers and mothers of these cross-eyed angels are trying in images of "depth" and "height" to express the deeper and higher dimensions of which these children are so often the messengers. The writers continuously give evidence not only of the special things that these people ask of them, but also of the gifts they give. One author looks at the fact that there's an excess of candidates for jobs as helpers and suggests that in all the idealism about caring for and protecting the weaker ones among us, there may be a little homesickness—a desire to escape to some place in the world where it is urgently required of you that you give the child in you room to run.

★   ★   ★

Worshiping with these children is a veritable festival. I was there last year at Christmas. You try, shyly at first, to join them, to be part of this world to which you belonged, long ago, when you weren't so grown up. Then you realize that it's more like coming home, and you try to get into the spirit of things. But fat volumes of dogmatics lie across your path, and you wonder with a bit of fear just who is really handicapped here. "Poor wretches!" said my neighbor, and I really got very angry when he said that. It's not usual to meet Christmas angels, cross-eyed or not.

★   ★   ★

One afternoon I chatted with the two priests there. They had just told, that Sunday, the story of the twelve-year-old Jesus who was first seen in the temple and then was brought home to the carpenter's shop, and then jokingly they told about their song in which the children pictured Jesus coming home to ask his mother for a sandwich. You see, they don't need our hymnbook. On the following Sunday, Jesus would make his way into the wider world, but not without singing an old Dutch tear-jerker: "Farewell, my dear parents, I'm leaving you now." On feast days they celebrate the Eucharist not with the usual wafers but with cake and soft drinks specially consecrated for the occasion. "We really cut big pieces of cake; it's a great feast, and we sing 'For He's a Jolly Good Fellow' to Jesus."

★   ★   ★

Let me tell you one more splendid story, about the time when the choir from Maria Roepaan sang in an ordinary parish church. They came to make it plain that "learning faith" is more real than "learning beliefs." In *A House Too Far?* the writers tell how the childen's reactions are not slowed down or adjusted by "marks of social polish."

On that particular Sunday morning it became clear all over again. The priest was serving communion, and the choir was singing. The priest was not at all sure whether the children in the choir would want to come for communion, too.

He thought they wouldn't. He assumed that they probably couldn't understand the mystery of Christ's presence. (And of course that was a sound assumption: who understands mysteries, anyhow?) So the priest walked solemnly over to the tabernacle to cover up the leftover hosts and then strode back to the altar. The choir finished its singing. And just as His Reverence started to say something, there came a voice from the choir: "Hey, you jackass, don't we get any?"

(2)

"What a feast, what a glorious feast," announced the minister. But as far as the eye could see (or the ear could hear), there was nothing to celebrate. And indeed, he said it in a voice of deadly seriousness, the servant of a dying church that had unlearned any lessons about making a feast, a man with more of trouble and torment in his sermon than of the kingdom. That he nevertheless spoke of a great feast came, it seemed to me, from the fact that the longing for a great celebration was still alive in him and that he was seeking to still that hunger with this fantasy.

★　★　★

The church of Maria Roepaan is no dying church. "We're the only one that's growing," says the priest. "A feast here every Sunday!" Deadly serious, rigid-faced people, unhappy because they quite mistakenly keep thinking that faith is something entirely above the eyebrows, learn there from retarded children how handicapped they themselves really are, how their originality, creativity, and spontaneity are all dammed up behind words that no longer say anything and rituals that no longer mediate anything. Herman Verbeek says, in *A Cup of Cold Water*, "Our liturgy has often become word play. Too much is demanded of our ears. The church makes its demands on our bottoms; liturgy is just an hour of sitting. You couldn't imagine anything more tedious. But a retarded child asks: Are you going to bring the drums today? Can we dance in a circle? Can we splash water? Who gets to light the candles? Will we have another feast next Sunday?" And many people in whom the longing for a feast is still alive learn to escape their stiffness from the children of Maria Roepaan and from the adults who can become "as little children." They clap their hands, dance around the altar after communion, give each other the kiss of peace, and create on the spot a new song of praise for creation, when the priest comes in with what looks like half of a produce market.

> Thank you for these lovely pears
> thank you for each lovely berry
> thank you, thank you hundredfold
> your creation makes us merry.

When I heard that song I remembered Missouri, where I sat down to dinner with a group of nuns in a convent. Before the meal we sat around the freshly set table with prayers full of confessions and suppressed depression, until a black woman, the only one present, suddenly made further prayer superfluous when she lifted her voice with merriment and devotion and prayed: "Thank you, Lord, for apple pie and whipped cream!"

The song of the pears and the berries, I admit, isn't going to make it into any new hymnbook. The text is thin; the rhyming is artificial; the melody is poor. But a mounting number of churchgoers come Sunday after Sunday through the rain, for they realize that their faith is freshened up by such a song. And I'd like for once to risk a pastoral/theological justification of the solo that one of the girls in the choir is allowed to sing. She has one leg. But in her song she's a cowboy, and on the four legs of her cow pony she races along across the prairie. That's her vision, *her* horse out of *her* revelation of how God makes all things new.

Hallelujah yippie-i-ay!

★ ★ ★

I'm listening to this song of longing with a retarded man of
about forty, who a year or so ago suddenly disappeared on
Easter Sunday afternoon. He was really nowhere to be found.
After a couple of hours the police called up. Was anyone
missing? They'd found the man shuffling along the highway
on the road to Nijmegen.

That evening he told his story. On this day, Easter Day,
Jesus was raised from the dead, but not Jesus alone—everyone! That's what Father had said. So he'd had to get to
Nijmegen, to the cemetery, for it was there that his parents
would arise, and of course they wouldn't know where to go, it
was so unexpected for them, and of course they'd want to see
him, and he them.

"He'd completely misunderstood the sermon, Father," said
the ward chief.

"Hah!" said the priest. "D'you think we understood it any
better?"

★ ★ ★

And what about consecrating cake and soft drinks on Jesus'
birthday? After all, "wine is soda for grownups," and cake and
soda mean a feast. I have some questions about that, of course,
but I don't dare ask them. Here I learn that I have much to
unlearn. But a moment later I heard myself asking a kind of
roundabout, cushion-shot question to communicate my
doubts about what the bishop thought of all this.

"We've never asked what the bishop thought. We always
ask our Lord directly, and so far he's approved of everything."

Anticipation

It was a couple of weeks before Christmas when he stepped
into my office in the clinic. An overgrown kid of twenty or so
who could only make contact with you by pushing at you

or pummeling you with his enormous hands; these marks of delicacy sometimes frightened me. He lifted a picture off the wall and asked me if he might have it.

"No," I said. "I'd rather keep it myself."

He pulled another picture off the wall. When I didn't appear willing to give that up, either, he ran over to my planter and yanked a plant out of it. "Then give me this." When I refused that, too, he kicked the plant across the room; clods of dirt flew everywhere. He was a prey to violent emotions.

Finally he sat down. "I've got to tell you something," he said. "I'm not coming to church at Christmastime. I'd just sit there blubbering with everybody around." And as stormily as he'd tumbled in, he disappeared. I still wanted to say something, but I was dumbfounded.

★   ★   ★

The mess in my office was more easily cleaned up than the confusion in my head and heart. What was really going on with that young man? He came to "get" something from me, but what? I wasn't sorry that I had protected my stuff, but what *could* I have *given* him? And why did I feel so guilty now?

I thought that maybe, with the intensity of his feelings, he'd revealed to me the poverty of my own feelings. Of course he'd revealed to me his own disturbed state, but by merely making that diagnosis I could get off the hook too easily. For alongside who *he* is, he was teaching me something about who *I* am. I'm somebody who reads the lines from Isaiah during Advent with his congregation:

> Oh, that Thou wouldst rend the heavens
> that Thou wouldst come down.
> that the mountains would tremble before Thy face
> as the flame sets dry twigs on fire
> as fire makes the water to boil over.

And I'm someone who at Christmas tells the old story of heavens rent asunder and a God who comes down and shepherds who were sore afraid; but I'm also someone to whom the intensity of those feelings of anticipation and fulfillment is unfamiliar.

What was it that was happening, not just in that boy but also in the shepherds, that they were so afraid? Shame? Guilt? Anxiety that they would come apart, the shivers at a new beginning, attachment to the darkness, deep emotion at discovering that God apparently knows you like the palm of his hand, fire in your dry twigs?

God knows.

★   ★   ★

Every year at Advent I have to think about that young man. And once I thought of him in the middle of summer. We were on the deck of a shrimp boat in the North Sea Canal just outside the Amsterdam harbor, awaiting the approach of the great windjammers that were celebrating the seven hundredth anniversary of the founding of the city. It was an overwhelming experience when there, not far from the Hem Bridge, a great three-masted ship under full sail loomed up in the mist. We waved and shouted, blew the ship's horn, and even felt a bit like crying: A ship! A ship with eight sails! The song of Jenny from Brecht's *Threepenny Opera* was borne in upon the wind:

> Now you gents all see I've the glasses to wash
> If a bed's to be made I make it.
> You may tip me with a penny, and I'll thank you very well
> And you see me dressed in tatters, and this tatty old hotel
> And you never ask how long I'll take it.
> But one of these evenings there will be screams from the harbor
> . . .
> And a ship with eight sails and
> All its fifty guns loaded
> Has tied up in the quay.

That woman was expecting great salvation.

★   ★   ★

When I ask people if they can tell me anything about their own anticipations at Christmastime, it seems that those expectations aren't very high. Living-room-sized. Warm companionship is much in demand. A few ask for more peace on earth, but without much conviction. Others ask for a new Christmas story, since we've gradually come to know what came to pass in those days all too well. The expectations aren't high, doomed in advance by the expectations of great evil in our days, and far afield from the sparkle with which Jenny in her tattered world looked forward to the day when there'd be screams from the harbor, and a great ship with eight sails and fifty guns loaded would tie up in the quay. Far afield, too, from the power with which Jews have dreamed of the future: rend the heavens asunder and come down! And far from the great shivers of the boy in my office, who in his own way came to tell me that if God should come near him it would be just too much for him.

★ ★ ★

What is going on when our expectations of salvation don't dare take on the dimensions of our expectations of evil? Who among us can speak to the question of his own expectations—I?—I wait for God himself—I expect that one day the mist will clear away and a ship will come, loaded to the brim!

Dreaming

The prisoner told me in all seriousness how an angel had appeared to him in the night, with a message about his wife and children. He wondered what his dream could mean and had had me summoned.

But I'm not Joseph.

I don't know how it is with you, but I always throw my dreams away immediately. Sometimes I'm ashamed of them; sometimes I'm afraid; sometimes I'm sorry that the dream is over; often the nonsense of it all surprises me; now and then the meaning of it comes to me. But in every case it's the same: a minute or two after I get up the dream's gone, and I won't see it again, for what the night brings is something I can't take with me into the day. You know, I preach about people to whom angels appeared in a dream with a message, but I myself don't see them, and they don't have any message for me. And if someone in prison comes to tell me he's seen them flying, I think: Su-u-u-u-u-re!

But which of us is really crazy?

I didn't have to think about that question for very long; it wasn't necessary for a messenger of God to appear to me in a dream to help me open my eyes. For there's a clear answer: I am crazy. I never paid any attention when the Bible describes how respectfully people dealt with their dreams, because they believed that it really could be that God would actually speak to them in their dreams. The patriarchs are said to have found consolation and inspiration in them, guidance for their lives. And Job says it well:

> In dreams, in visions of the night,
> when deepest sleep falls upon men,
> while they sleep on their beds,
> God makes them listen.

But the theologians have no ears for this; they maintain a stony silence, and so they avoid any disagreements about it. They're all in agreement: whether once upon a time the angels really scrambled up and down or whether that's only (!) a stylistic medium of the storyteller makes little difference; anyone these days who thinks that God uses dreams as a means of communication needs to head straight for the doctor's office.

But when psychotherapists know how human beings can come to healing through dreams, can set things right with themselves, their spouses, their children, and God: can theologians then simply ignore the possibility that people can come to redemption through dreams? And if people say that it is God who has called to them in the night, called to them to awake and to arise from the dead, may theologians then say, "Sorry, but you're mistaken. That was no doubt once the case with Jacob and Joseph and Samuel, but since Freud and Jung we see such things a bit differently, you know. It all has to do with the unconscious, you see, and dreaming is not a supernatural, divine reality, but a natural, human one"?!

When Peter climbs to the roof of the house of Simon the tanner and has a vision there, certainly there are natural reasons for it. Peter is confronted by the then vital question: What to do about non-Jews who want to become Christians? What about the Jewish dietary laws, for example? Are they still valid? Of course they are! Or are they? Peter is at the point of transition from old to new, and he himself has no idea what to do. So it is time for prayer.

It's around noontime. In order to pray Peter retires to the flat roof under the heavens. Cooking smells waft up from the house below, tickling Peter's nose. He prays. Then he has a vision. He dreams of . . . eating. A sheet descends from heaven, on it many kinds of animals. Peter's a Jew; he knows the dietary laws. There's a difference between clean and unclean. On the sheet he sees unclean animals. And a voice says, "Rise up, Peter, kill and eat!" Peter resists. God, no! I've never eaten such things. Unclean!

The voice again: "What God has called clean you may not consider unclean."

Peter is speechless. He . . .

But the voice comes a third time. (It isn't the first occasion when Peter's been addressed three times.) Then the curtain falls on the dream. While Peter, up on the roof, is not tossing the dream aside but is trying to puzzle out its meaning, two unclean pagans are knocking on the door downstairs. Peter stands up. And now the gospel goes out into the *whole* world. "For God has caused me to see . . ." says Peter.

Or did you think that it was Peter himself who caused Peter to see?

Forget it! You're dreaming!

Panizza

A machine had indicated that the man had a small spot on his lung, so he landed in our hospital. *Cancer* is the first thought that pops up in the mind of such a poor fellow when he hears that kind of message, and mostly that's right.

I went to visit him.

"I'm the minister," I said.

"That can't be," he answered.

My astonished look told him I needed clarification. "I'm just an ordinary workman," he said.

I sat down, and slowly his sad story came out. I could sum it up this way: "You feel that at particular moments in your life the church has left you in the lurch."

Yes, that was so.

I promised to come back soon. Here was a job to do.

He looked at me suspiciously. "You mean that?" he asked. Then he repeated, "I'm just an ordinary worker."

I answered that naturally I'd give first preference to the rich folks, but I hoped there would be some time left over for him. Fortunately, he bought this.

A day or so later I was with him again, and he continued his unhappy story, but without so much grumbling about the church. He seemed ready to go a layer deeper; this time he was talking about how at certain moments *God* had left him in the lurch. He thought of himself as a "poor" man over against "rich" men, to whom God did pay attention, to whom God did give happiness and faith. He grew angry about a God who has made it so terribly complicated to believe in him, who has invented such godawful filthy sicknesses, and who in any case doesn't extend a helping hand when a poor bugger who doesn't deserve it is pounced on by one of them.

I wanted to say something, but he was clearly so afraid that I'd speak up for the so-called Almighty that he immediately snubbed me. "Please don't come around with your eyewash, because you people don't know Thing One about it. Just let me rot here, and don't you try to talk me into heaven, because I don't want any of it."

★   ★   ★

I had to think about him again when I saw the portrayal of heaven in Oskar Panizza's play *The Council of Love*. Those images are still on my retinas days afterward. God is a degenerate, physically and spiritually incontinent man, who asks the Devil to think up something nasty to punish the human beings below for their evil. The Devil then gets a lovely inspiration: send an utterly beautiful woman to earth as the carrier of syphilis. Mary, Ever Virgin, is absolutely thrilled. Obviously, that person herself has a dubious sex life hidden in her past somewhere, and she gets a kick out of thinking how the people down there will soon be caught out.

Jesus is present, too, a chip off the old block, a half-baked, effeminate type who nods his head assiduously when God tells the Devil that he agrees, but only on condition that the human race will keep longing for redemption, because otherwise that'll be the end of the heavenly business.

How did Panizza come to such a picture of God? In a speech in his own defense (of course he was accused of blasphemy, you'd already guessed that!), he said that this profile was provided to him by the church and its servants. And he trounced this church and its servants in the scenes that take place on earth. They were set in the papal court, where the courtiers theologize, moralize, and dogmatize far from suffering human beings amidst corrupt cardinals and posturing courtesans.

I saw this play in the town of 's-Hertogenbosch, in the theater next to St. John's Cathedral. The auditorium was full of believers and former believers. I found it difficult to gauge their reactions, but I am inclined to suppose that this happening furthered the community's spiritual health in this bishop's city and its surroundings, because this play put words and images to the anger about the bitter mystery of suffering and pain. Perhaps it helped, too, because it tried to deal with the theology of retribution and with the kind of theology that taught retribution, and with the church that for convenience' sake forbade us to think and told us to keep away from a number of feelings, particularly sexual and aggressive feelings.

The anger of Catholics and former Catholics, says the psychologist of religion Father Willem Berger, appears in two ways: "No one will put up any longer with a church that presents a God who alienates and who tries to persuade me to sell my soul. But also no one wants a God who in one way or another extradites me to the church which mediated the selling of my soul."

★ ★ ★

Oskar Panizza wrote his play in 1894. He was sentenced to a year in prison. After his release he was a broken man. He tried to get admitted to an institution, but they wouldn't have him. He tried to hang himself but got cold feet at the last moment. One day in 1904 he ran through the streets of Munich wearing only a shirt. He was picked up and put in an institution, where he died in 1921.

He is now in heaven.

Francis

It has been 750 years since Francis, with his brothers and with Sister Death, celebrated dying, and I wanted to devote a few thoughts to that. But you have to be careful about it. I realized that all over again after a recent worship service in the prison, which I'd wanted to begin with a prayer of the poor little brother. "You'd better put that out of your head," said a prisoner.

"You don't think it'd be a good idea if I prayed that prayer of Saint Francis with you?"

"No, I don't. You'd better stay away from it."

"You think it's a holier prayer than I have a right to have on my lips?"

"Your suit's too nice—and how much are you earning here with us this morning?"

Conversation was difficult. I had to exert all my efforts not to flip over into countertransference by getting defensive or aggressive. Besides, some people in the church were getting rebellious; they'd come for a worship service, not a debate. I wondered if I should leave the ninety-and-nine in the sheepfold while I went searching for the one, but I decided that wasn't a good plan.

"Reverend, can't we get rid of him?"

I said that I felt uncertain, but that I knew one thing for sure:

I didn't want him to get out. I said that we all have a tendency to get "jamming transmitters" out of the way, whether they were rogues or saints, by putting them in cells or niches, and that they knew better than I did how disastrous that way often is. I remembered suddenly how Saint Francis was buried on a hill where once criminals had been buried in unconsecrated ground. And I said that I hoped that we, in this consecrated place, could give one another a bit of room, with respect for one another and for Saint Francis, and for the Lord he pictured for us with his surprising images, both for rogues and for solid citizens. But I said it too clumsily, I think, for people didn't seem to listen too well, and the original objector took on the role of a victim and disappeared. Anyhow, I got the feeling that he took Francis out with him and in any case I tried a different prayer.

★ ★ ★

In the town archives of Assisi they have found a document that tells in detail how one carried out the banishment of those who then were the most rejected of human beings: the lepers. Several people have seen in that document how outrageously the church compromised itself by this merciless "good riddance" full of devotional God-talk and pious ceremomial, but I experience it rather differently, and I even think that we can learn something from it.

This is the bewildering ritual. The priest comes out of the sacristy and goes to the place where the person who has become a leper is kneeling, segregated from the faithful. He sprinkles the leper with holy water and says, "Beloved poor one of God, by means of great affliction and torment, sickness, leprosy, and many vicissitudes humans can earn the kingdom of heaven, where there will be no more sickness and sorrow and all is pure and clean, without spot or wrinkle, more sparkling than the sun. You shall come there if God pleases. . . . My Brother, the separation applies only to your body. As pertains to your spirit—and this is more important—you remain as before a participant in the prayers of our Mother, the holy Church, as if you were attending the Mass in person daily. Loving people will care for your lesser needs and God will never abandon you. Amen."

The celebrant sprinkles earth taken from the nearby churchyard upon the head of the sick person and says: "Die to the world so that you may be born anew of God. O Jesus, my savior, who formed me from the earth and clothed me with a body, grant that I may be raised again in the last day." The congregation answers: "My bones shake and my soul flows out from within me. Hallelujah. Be gracious unto us, O God, and deliver us from evil."

The gospel is read, the story of the ten lepers. Then follow the instructions: "My brother, take this mantle as a symbol of humility, and do not go out without wearing it. In the name of the Father, and of the Son, and of the Holy Ghost.

"Take this cup and receive in it whatever is given you to drink; and as a matter of obedience, I forbid you to drink from rivers, fountains, or springs.

"If upon your way you should encounter any person who wishes to speak with you, then I forbid you to answer him until you have turned your face into the wind.

"It is forbidden to you to speak with any woman, unless she be your wife. It is forbidden to you to visit churches or chapels or to go to a mill or a marketplace. Never may you travel on narrow streets where people cannot avoid you. Take this rattle and with it warn others of your approach."

Then the procession is organized to accompany the leper to his new dwelling. A wooden cross is installed on the door. The leper says, "Here is my permanent resting place. Here shall I live. This is my promise."

In front of the door stands a poor box. The priest makes the first contribution, and after him all the faithful. They return to the church, but the leper remains behind. "Almighty God, who by the sufferings of thy Son hast conquered the arrogance of the ancient Enemy, give to thy servant the power to endure with patience and devotion the evil that has come upon him. Amen."

And the people answer, "Amen."

Saint Francis has said that the turning point of his life was on the road from Maria Angelica to Foligno, where he met a leper, a stinking, repulsive tramp. He throws him a few coins and spurs his horse onward. But suddenly he "sees" that in this leper God himself is holding out his hand to him. Then Francis jumps from his horse, kneels by the leper, takes his hand, and kisses it.

Anybody who's wearing a nice suit and living securely really has to be quite careful with such a story.

Pain

"We're going out riding in the carriage for the whole day! A magical sound that brings the spirits of my brothers and sisters (not to speak of my own) to a state of ecstasy, almost a blessed frenzy. Out for the whole day!"

So runs a childhood memory of François Haverschmidt, Dutch poet and minister of the nineteenth century. A few moments later he exclaims, "Heavens, how beautiful the earth is on such a summer's day!"

But then the story takes a sharp turn.

"Odd, but while the others go on singing I suddenly get lost in thought about the question which of us shall have to die first. I go down the whole list, one by one: father, mother, my oldest brother, my middle brother, my youngest sister, finally my baby brother, and I come to the conclusion that I can't do without any of them.

"And secretly I say a little prayer that if anyone has to die soon, it'll be me, or else (for, after all, I can see a lot of arguments against that, too) and perhaps preferably, my aunt! The simpleton!

"Imagine her knowing what is being asked 'on her behalf' in her immediate vicinity, right while she's bending over me and mother is whispering her opinion that I must certainly have fallen asleep because I'm so quiet."

★ ★ ★

I've always loved that story, and I have to think of it often when I'm happy with other people in a land of milk and honey, and all of a sudden something shifts inside, and I know that all this will pass away, and the joy over what's good and lovely gets all mixed with the bitterness that it is all fragile and will break.

I've always loved that story, but I certainly keep my love for it under wraps. You're not supposed to show your sadness too much, and you're not supposed to cherish it, and you have to be very careful with it. François Haverschmidt finally did himself in; he was so hung up about this question of life and death that he could cope with it only by hanging himself.

But now, in a week when I am experiencing a great deal of grief, I've gotten a meditation on grief from a priest, and it's really something to chew on.

★ ★ ★

He speaks of grief as a dark "figured bass" that runs beneath the melody of life. You have to accept its right to exist, he says. And you mustn't be ashamed of the fact that as a believer you can nonetheless be sad deep within. You don't have to fall into a black melancholy in order to say that human life isn't possible without grief and sadness. If you venture into life, you get wounded. If you love someone, you will weep over that person. Love wants to be stronger than death, and tries to keep death away from the beloved; but Verhoeven rightly says that that effort is always going to be accompanied by the sorrowful awareness that it is doomed to failure.

That's why I recently talked at a wedding about love and faithfulness "until death us do part," mentioning both the beauty and the pain of that. There were those who thought that I shouldn't have said that. I shouldn't have brought that up in church. But I think the church is especially the place where you can consider such things. "Melancholy is a hallmark of human authenticity," says Verhoeven. It's not black depression but a gentle sorrow that really belongs in life when we look at it honestly. And if I believe that the gospel is a light that shines in the darkness, then I don't have to deny the darkness. Because if I do, then the light serves no purpose whatever.

★ ★ ★

And if someone asks about that light, then I have to say something about the Man of Sorrows, who does not take my sorrows away but who does tell me not to be broken by them; he has already done that. I don't have to finish something that he's already finished. And sadness doesn't have the last word.

But in the meantime the gospel does not yet wipe the tears from my eyes. I still cry my heart out at a loss. But I prick up my ears when somewhere a humble servant of our Lord reminds himself and me of the promises in the Book that the tears shall be wiped away.

And what else?

Ton Lemaire wrote a wonderful book about tenderness, which consoles because it can reconcile one with one's own vulnerability, and with the fact that everything, everything shall pass away. The last sentence of that book reads: "Let us be gentle with one another, for life is unbearable pain."

Gary Gilmore

People who know that I worked in a psychiatric clinic for prisoners in America and that I visited prisons in Kansas want to know what I think about the execution of Gary Gilmore, the double murderer, who was put to death in Utah by a firing squad.

I don't know what I think about that.

It is, of course, a scandal before God and humankind; that's clear. The American psychiatrist Karl Menninger judges this in his book *The Crime of Punishment* as a "crime against a criminal." And no doubt it was fair that churches and social action groups stood protesting in front of the gates of that hell in Utah.

Still I don't know if I'd have taken part in such an action.

As far as I am concerned, the problem is not so much one of capital punishment, although many people feared that after this first carrying out of a death sentence in ten years, more would quickly follow. In my estimation, the question is one of euthanasia.

★   ★   ★

I still remember very well an interview with a pitiful black man who had two life sentences in the state prison at Lansing, Kansas. "Will he ever get out?" I asked the guard, at the same time realizing that I'd asked a dead-end question.

How does such a person, ill-prepared anyway, live in such a jungle, with a past but no future? To get at answers that would escape the ordinary stereotypes, we worked out the following question: "Imagine this prison as a person, a human being. What would that person look like?"

He answered immediately, "Like an old man, a blind old man."

"And what is that blind old man doing?"

"Waiting."

"For what?"

"For nothing."

★   ★   ★

Gary Gilmore didn't want to wait for nothing any longer. He was thirty-six years old, and for exactly half that time he had lived in institutions and prisons. A brief love affair with an equally unstable woman gave him for a moment the hope that something good might happen for him, but when she broke off the affair his whole world caved in. That was the day he died, I think, and whatever there was left of him wandered around aimlessly for a few days, killed two innocent people, and was arrested and sentenced to death.

"Let's do it," said Gilmore, to everyone's astonishment. "It's a good sentence."

Completely within the power of that blind old man, Gary Gilmore could only make something out of his life by making something out of his death. For his life he could no longer count on any kind of help, but for his death he could. Suicide with the assistance of five riflemen.

But not every suicide is the desperate behavior of a shattered human being. Not every suicide is a spiritual failure. R. F.

Diekstra says in a study that suicide is not always self-murder, but can also be the ending of bodily life so as to save the self. "There are people who commit suicide in order to accomplish things that are very important for them."

In that light I think it may be a good thing that people took Gilmore seriously when he asked them in so many words to keep their hands off his death.

One more thing . . .

Just before the execution the prison chaplain laid his hand on Gilmore's shoulder. But it was Gilmore who uttered the priestly words: *"Dominus vobiscum."* The Lord be with you. Why the Latin?

Words from an earlier time, from believing like a little child?

Holy words, because everyday language has been befouled and can't express the mystery?

I immediately had to think of the inmate who urged me to say (in the Christmas service) "Unto us a child is born" in Latin, because otherwise Christmas wouldn't be real, and he was moved by hearing that news from on high. *Puer nobis natus est.*

Of that Child it is said that he suffered—was crucified next to murderers—died—descended into hell—on the third day arose from the dead—and ascended into heaven. All of that must have been a part of what was said when the priest answered Gilmore, *"Et cum spiritu tuo."* And with thy spirit.

Senile

The nurses are bringing in the old people. Senile old people. We've turned a room into a chapel, and we're going to have a worship service. Some of them are sitting in wheelchairs or are rolled in on their beds. Others shuffle in under their own power. Some of them become confused and are shown to a chair. "My carriage awaits; I have to go," says one. "In a minute," I reply. "First let's sing and pray."

Someone yells that he wants his hat back. A nurse says that you can't sit in church with a hat on, but he keeps protesting.

"Old bitch!" he says. A woman from Pavilion Two is sitting there beaming at me and humming "Silent Night." We often sing it for her, even in the middle of summer. I give out the song sheets for the hymns we're going to sing, the hit parade of yesteryear. "A Mighty Fortress." "Onward Christian Soldiers." "Rock of Ages."

"I won't sing," someone announces angrily. Another keeps repeating sadly, "I don't have any money with me."

"Who are you?" asks a woman I've known for years. As a child, she worked in a stone factory, and she can tell a heart-rending story about that. It is in fact the only story left in her repertoire.

There are strange boarders at our Lord's table, and these are the strangest. I put on my robe, light the candles. "Our help is in the name of . . ." But I feel helpless. How did I get started in all this? I can still hear the burned-out doctor saying, "They're all ripe for the disposal chute," his feelings so overwhelming that he had to hide behind a wall of cynicism. "Mad as hatters, all of them." Yes, it's true, but they're still children of God. They may forget everything else, but not that, if possible.

We sing. "Abide with Me." Right up front there sits a deaf woman. She can't hear a word, but if I go over and sing right into her ear, she gets the knack of it. "Help of the helpless, O abide with me."

★　★　★

And I preach. Wonder if they understand any of it. It seems to me that they don't. But as I see it, that's not important, for I imagine that something of God's peace that passes all understanding comes down to them as I tell the mysterious stories of our faith and let them hear the deep words, the old words that lead you into green pastures. For example:

"Here's the sermon. It's about being afraid. When I was a little boy I was often afraid. And I thought, when I grow up, I won't be afraid anymore. Now I'm grown up, and I'm still afraid sometimes, just like before.

"Back then I was often afraid that my father and mother had abandoned me. I'd wake up with a start in the middle of the night. And I'd call out. Then my mother would come and sit on the edge of my bed. And she'd tell me a story, or we'd sing a song.

"Now we're in church. We're all frightened people. So I'll tell a story and we'll sing a song. We won't sing 'We Are Not Afraid.' That's a street song for frightened people. We'll sing 'We *Are* Afraid.' That's a song of faith for faithful people. They're also scared people, of course, but because they have faith, they believe that they can do something about being afraid. They believe that they can go to each other with it, and together to God. They believe that God can do something about it.

"Fear can be big, big as a giant, big as Goliath. It can get to you in your dreams, too. Dreams that a giant will get you. I used to dream a lot that I fell into the water. I sank down and sank down and cried out. But I was lost; nobody heard me. I think I dreamed that I was going to die all alone. That was scary. How happy I was when I woke up and saw my own room again. And I knew that in the next room there was no giant, and no evil stepmother, but a king and a queen: my father and mother.

"You can't do much about fear. It comes just as scary dreams come. There isn't any protection against it. You can't say, well, I'll put on my armor, and the fear won't be able to get through. It gets through anyway.

"Jesus was also very scared. It's completely human. You can't get around it. But faith says that you *can* get through it. God keeps seeing you. And you need to keep seeing God. If you've just got a little bit of faith, as little as that stone of David's, you can make it. The fear is still there, but now it's different. You look at it differently; you see it differently. You believe that story told by Mother Church, that God, like your Father, won't let you go. On the other side of death's dark night God is waiting. God is there when you wake up, the King!

"Do you know who also believed that? Luther. He was a brave man, but sometimes he too was scared. It got very dark around him then. Do you know what he did? He took a piece of chalk and he wrote on his slate three words: *I've been baptized.*

I'm not alone. Even if I *feel* abandoned, without a father and a mother, a little boy in a big dark woods where there are wild beasts, I believe something else. I believe . . . how shall I say it? I believe that I can't be drowned in the deep waters. I've been *through* the deep waters. I've been baptized. And God called me by name, and there's a promise:

> Jesus loves me! this I know,
> For the Bible tells me so.
> Little ones to Him belong,
> We are weak, but He is strong.

"Amen."

★ ★ ★

We sing a few more songs. I try a silent prayer. It's utterly quiet. I give the benediction. I collect the song sheets. I shake hands. Someone is crying. Others show no reaction at all. One woman thanks me. "You're such a darling," she says. One man says he didn't get a worship sheet, but I know he's got it hidden under his vest and I fish it out. I may be a darling, but I'm not stupid.

"Will we have church again soon?"

"Here's your hat back," says the nurse.

"We didn't sing 'How Great Thou Art.' "

And then, of course, there's that man in the wheelchair with his inevitable "Reverend, I don't have any money with me." He hasn't long to live, I know. Soon he'll roll off to heaven's gates. And once again he'll say, but then, we may trust, for the last time, "I don't have any money with me."

Breath

For a moment I thought he was dead, stillborn, our oldest son, when he lay there so motionless that first second, but all of a sudden a trembling shot through that little body, air whistled into his lungs, the first breath, a scream of fright. And just as when you're the witness of someone's last breath, something like a prayer runs through you, when God's breath moves upon the face of the waters and breathes into a human being the breath of life, or takes it back again.

I have to think about that sometimes, the breath of God and the breath of a human being. I work in a lung clinic, where so many suffer and die breathlessly. The whole creation groans, sighs; it is so terrifying, so breathtaking.

★   ★   ★

In books I've read how a child gets its breath, as it were, from its mother. The first cry after a birth is indeed a scream of fright, and no wonder. You are roughly thrust from the warm security of mother's body. "You do it all by yourself now," said our "world-famous humble country doctor," severing our son's umbilical cord. It was said very matter-of-factly. Imagine! All of a sudden, within the next second, you have to breathe for yourself. "Quiet now, you don't have to get into the world yet," the writer Annie Schmidt has a mother say to the fruit of her womb, but the moment comes when you do have to get into it, and the sudden loneliness and freedom give you a fit. You scream about that, and at the very moment you draw your first breath, fear of the void nearly chokes you to death.

But if father and mother rock the child in their arms and hum to it that all is good (and behold, it was very good, the first day), then the little thing can recover its breath. And it will be the same on the following days—and weeks, and months—the weak and often uneven breathing of the child becomes relaxed, develops in parallel with the restful breathing of the mother. And with coos and shrieks, the child will answer her, responding to the breathing of her voice.

Unfortunately, just the opposite can also happen: anxious mothers (who, for example, can accept the child or themselves only with difficulty, unfree women whose breathing itself is unfree) cannot assure their children that everything is good, behold, very good. The breath catches in their throats, and that might be contagious. They are bent down under life's load, and from the beginning the child sighs with them. The great spaces make the child insecure, and the child "holds his breath." The doctor has to come. And sometimes has to keep coming.

★ ★ ★

And in the Book of books I read how a human being gets its breath from God. Through his Word the heavens are made, all their host through the breath of his mouth, says the psalmist. God's breath moved over the waters, and he breathed the breath of life into Adam's nose. Just as it's the mother who gives the child her breath and in doing so places it in the world and calls it to freedom, so also God creates humankind by giving it breath, his breath. And God's Word, his articulated breath, tells us that all is good, behold, very good, and even when I have to walk through the valley of the shadow of death, I will fear no evil. Life is breathed into humankind through the breath of God, and since we were in our cradles God, who from our mother's arms, hath helped us on our way with countless gifts of love, still is ours today.

★ ★ ★

The breathing of the child will never reach adulthood unless it is accompanied by mother's word of goodness and peace. A child that must do without its mother's comfort and warmth will often die or live out its life in anxiety. Human freedom is made possible by love of the one who gives freedom.

At Pentecost, dead and unfree and anxious people get to hear the message that they can breathe easy and are born again. "Peace be with you!" said Jesus. "And after saying this, he breathed on them and said, 'Receive the Holy Breath.' " And his friends came to life at the breath of his voice. And behold, it was good, and the breath was articulated in words, and the word was understandable in every tongue.

"As one whom his mother comforts, so will I comfort you," God had said. The Comforter has come. The physician sent by God has restored the disturbed relationship.

Millstone

In prison he was submissiveness itself, but in his family he must have been a tyrant. Learned people know that this double picture is seen often enough and that both kinds of behavior serve to mitigate the feeling of uncertainty that is experienced in contacts between people.

Contacts between people were, by the way, what had gotten the man into a terrible fix, for he was caught in an incestuous relationship with his daughter. Daughter to an institution, father to jail, and mother back home with the rest of the children. As a way of healing a sick family system it's poor, but that's not what I want to discuss just now. I want to discuss the man. There was almost no sign of life in him any longer; he seemed to have become completely silent. His fellow prisoners, honest thieves, denounced him as a child rapist. He kept them at some distance by exaggerating the difference in their ages. ("Those young men don't know what they're talking about, or what life's all about, and they don't have enough respect for their elders.") At the same time he was silently communicating the message that he was too old to change.

In all kinds of colleges nowadays, students are taught that a person can change only if he himself believes in change, but perhaps they'll accept my word that you can also believe on someone else's behalf. But in that case you really should have some hope in the house and not get discouraged too soon.

★   ★   ★

For the first few months there was no movement to be seen in the man. "Just stay where you are and don't budge" was his message, as if he were playing a game of Statues. He even had a Bible text to justify his stubbornness; such a thing is always suspect, I think, but in this case it was completely so, because the man was Catholic. "What are you yammering about?" he said. "That Jesus of yours said himself that whoever causes a child to sin should have a millstone placed around his neck and be thrown into the depths of the sea." Tautly and with a kind of triumph, he watched this shot to see if it would hit the mark.

"What do you think of that?" he asked.

"Rather good," I said stonily.

What was it that Rabbi Bunam used to teach?

The great guilt of human beings is not created by the sins they commit: temptation is great and our powers are small. The great guilt is that when we *can* repent, we don't.

I ran across the same intriguing thought in the work of the American theologian Charles Curran, who said that the sin of Judas was not his betrayal of Christ but his terrible, violent self-condemnation.

What's going on in our man sitting there weighed down and immovable in his punishment corner with that millstone around his neck, given to him by our Lord Jesus himself as a mark of rejection? Self-condemnation? Anxiety? Impotence?

But after several months there gradually came a little sign of life, of faith. Very carefully some contacts with his children were arranged. Some of them came now and then to visit him.

★ ★ ★

Several more months went by. The time for his release was approaching. He went to live in a rented apartment, found a job. Gallantly he tried to get involved in life a little bit. Things didn't go too badly. But then he saw his vacation coming, and that scared him. If you can't live the time well, you have to kill time, and that's dreadful work.

About then, I had to visit someone in the Detention Center in Maastricht, and I asked him if he'd like to go for a ride. It was around the end of his vacation.

"What have you been doing?" I asked.

"Nothing" was what I expected him to say.

"I spent a day in Den Bosch," he said. He gave me his what-do-you-think-of-that look, but this time there was a spark of fun in his eyes.

"What did you do there?" I asked.

"I went to St. John's Cathedral," he said. He told me about it, fascinated by the faith of the people who had thought up that church, and built it. Of course, one can pray anywhere, but in a place like that it's somehow easier to fall on your knees.

But. He had gone to the altar dedicated to Mary. Men and women were kneeling there. He'd looked at them. He'd wanted to kneel, too, but couldn't. He'd wanted to get a candle and light it with a little prayer, just as he'd done when he was a boy. Quite simple, really. Candle, kneel, pray. But he hadn't been able to do it.

He was very sad when he told me about that. "Dumb!" he said, "not to be able to do what you used to. Just ordinary prayer. Like the other people there."

I didn't know what to say. Such a good story! Such a brave confession! When he was still a child, he behaved as a child, prayed as a child. But when he became a man he became a tyrant. And a submissive servant. He'd put aside childish things.

Tyrants and submissive servants can't pray. Indeed, I tell you, unless ye become as little children . . .

★   ★   ★

A short while later he told still another story. "I made another little excursion," he said.

"Where'd you go?"

"To the Open-air Bible Museum at the Holy Land Foundation."

"How was that?"

"Beautiful." He told me about it. Just the way a father would tell a child, I thought, and I told him that, too.

"Y'know what I also saw there?" he asked, after a silence.

"No, what?" I said.

"A millstone."

"How'd it look?"

"Big."

"What did you do with it?"

"I . . . I left it there."

"So you thought, just let it lie there, in the Holy Land." He smiled. He looked very cheerful.

Then he gave me a poke in the ribs and said, "You turkey!"

Weary Wanderer

My grandfather was a minister on the island of Urk. A Dutch nursery rhyme tells about a minister from Urk who had to preach on the island of Schokland but forgot his sermon because the movement of the boat made him seasick. Well, that was *not* my grandfather! For born and bred in Elburg, this fisher of men always remained something of a fisherman. He'd wanted to go to sea, but he was turned down—and just about the same time his father got religion.

His father, my great-grandfather, was the music master in Elburg. Even though he was not a man of faith but very much a man of the world who liked his shot of gin and didn't mind his wife smoking cigarillos, he'd nevertheless become a church organist and played when the psalms were sung on Sundays there by the side of the Zuider Zee.

One time the minister got sick. With a great deal of difficulty they finally managed to get an evangelist. In those days the Salvation Army was coming up in the world, and obviously the evangelist had been inspired by that merry movement. What happened after the sermon on that Sunday is still talked about in Elburg. The evangelist called for a song:

Come, says Jesus' holy word
From your night shall you be stirred
Come, you shall from fear be free,
Weary wanderer, come to me.

But the organ was silent. When a second call for the revival song also remained unanswered, the evangelist himself climbed up to the balcony where the organ keyboard stood. There was my great-grandfather kneeling by the organ bench in tears.

"That weary wanderer," he said. "That's me. Will you pray with me?"

★ ★ ★

"A powerful conversion," they said in Elburg. On that very same day my great-grandfather sent off a telegram to America, where two of his children, because of his poverty, were being reared by a rich sister, with the exhortation to bend their knees before Jesus, too.

And those who sat on a bench after a walk along the town ramparts could always tell where ter Linden had been sitting: with his walking stick he had written in the sand, "Jesus loves you, too."

You can come to faith in Elburg, but you can fall away from it, too. That's what happened to my grandmother's brother, who escaped from Gloomyburg (as he liked to call it) to live a worldly life in Amsterdam. Exactly what he was up to I don't know. My grandmother, worried about his eternal salvation, refused (to my considerable regret) to give out any details about his life and times. All I know is that, whatever it was, he needed a dinner jacket for it, and I've worn that jacket for years with pleasure. So, although I never knew him (too bad!), there's a special way in which I always feel a bond with him.

When my grandfather was turned down for a career at sea, his father asked him if he didn't want to become a minister. He did. And he did become one, but always right by the water: Urk, Langweer, and Amsterdam. He could tell great stories, particularly about Urk. There was blind Jelle, or the two servant girls who both used the very same set of false teeth, or the fisherman who told him at his installation that he should pretend he was standing there talking to a bunch of cabbages.

In Langweer he felt like a missionary. In an interview after his retirement, he said, "I was able to start all kinds of societies, singing societies in particular, for with singing you can reach many people. Music has great power."

In 1910 my grandfather left for Amsterdam. "After Langweer I figured that I'd find a lot more knowledge in churchly Amsterdam. What a disenchantment it was when I asked in a catechism class who the first man was and the answer came back, 'Luther!' "

★ ★ ★

On October 4, 1943, my grandfather took his leave of Amsterdam. He did so in the Westerkerk. As he came in, the organist played the melody of Grandfather's favorite song.

87

Come, says Jesus' holy word
From your night shall you be stirred
Come, you shall from fear be free,
Weary wanderer, come to me.

And my grandfather was deeply moved when he mounted the
stairs into the pulpit for the last time.

★ ★ ★

Next Sunday I shall, for the *first* time, mount those stairs.
Amsterdam is no longer a churchly town. Adam is no longer
the "first man." Our organist, Simon C. Jansen, has never
heard of the hymn about the weary wanderer. But singing and
Jesus' holy word still have great power.

A Little Pastoral Word List

After having worked for several years in hospitals and
prisons, I've returned to the bosom of the church. With
mixed feelings, for as I crossed the threshold again I put
myself at a distance from many who don't feel at home there.
Those people have meant a lot for me and for my faith; you
meet genuine people there, often spiritually gifted and
respectfully dealing with the basic issues of life. Such people
could mean a lot to the church, but the church no longer
means anything much to them. Because things have gotten
too rigid. Because faith is frozen in words and rites in which
nothing happens anymore and in which we hide ourselves
from the voice of the living God. Or because we know too
much about God. Or because we have shrunk the gospel to
its *social* relevance. Or because that relevance, by and large,
does *not* come into view. Or because all the mystery and the
trembling are gone out of it; the liturgy is heavy and flat;
there's no holy playing to do, nothing to refresh yourself
with. Or because your emotional life withers and runs flat.
Ah, so many people!
I'm going to miss those people a lot.

★ ★ ★

And especially I'll miss their directness, and particularly the directness of the inmates of the Pompekliniek, a psychiatric institution for the treatment of people who have committed one or more serious crimes. Their inner emotional brakes are defective, and they also can't use the "brakes" society puts on them through law and custom, so they often have their hearts right behind their tongues; whatever comes to mind, they offer it to you unfiltered. The moment you show up on the ward and are identified to them as a pastor, the stereotypes get trotted out. The priest and I once made a list of the thoughts that spontaneously came up whenever we appeared, and then we sat there musing about what they might mean.

One of my American teachers had a way of handling similar situations. When he was sitting in an airplane, and the person next to him got into a conversation with him and asked him what he did for a living, he would of course admit that he belonged to our Lord's ground crew. The pause that almost invariably ensued he would handle by saying with a smile, "That makes you kind of uncomfortable, eh?"

If it's true that in prison chaplaincy you see the same things that you'd see in an ordinary parish, but as if through a magnifying glass, then those first reactions to the chaplain on the part of prisoners in the clinic are indications of what happens in silence and in the hearts of less spontaneous mortals when they meet ministers and priests.

From our collection I'll pull out the best ones.

★　★　★

To begin with, there are the immediate associations with the collection of money and resistance to that.

"Nope, Father, nothing to collect here; try the Vatican."

"You can't collect anything from me, Reverend. You know, that Boss of yours didn't even have a stone to lay his head on. If you want something, try the rich folks."

It's never simple to find a good response to things like that, but sometimes you luck out and get past the resistance to the underlying thoughts and feelings. As often as not you run up against bitterness: bitterness against churches and people who should be living unselfishly but don't do so either. "Everything is corrupt; this whole world revolves around money, booze, and broads—it's an illusion to believe that it's any better anywhere, that anywhere there is a chance of real rest, that there's really any decent place in this rotten world. Nope, you can forget all that crap."

Behind *that* often enough lies bitterness about their own lives, about the difficulty they have in avoiding being caught up with "money, booze, and broads," or in being able to live freer, more generous, less care-laden lives, like the birds of the air and the lilies of the field.

I think of the man who would behave horribly toward women and girls, but who at the same time had a deep devotion to the Virgin Mary. His misfortune, his sin, his sickness—whatever you want to call it—was that he couldn't get the two closer together. A woman as a partner was unknown to him. For him she was a creature of the gutter and he didn't even know her name, or else he put her on a pedestal and hallowed her name. As a sign of contempt, he always called me "Paisley," as if I were that Irishman who represents a church that refuses to give Mary the honor which is her due.

To the priest he used to say, "Listen, I use whores, but I sure as hell had better never catch you doing it."

In all of that I hear a longing for a little holy ground nearby, a desire to live there, and a complete lack of faith that it will ever happen.

★ ★ ★

"Heaven" is another association. Many people feel called to let you know right after you get there that dead is dead and heaven a fairy tale. "After all, nobody ever came back from there, and besides, it'd become too full. No, you won't make me believe that."

"Make me more of a believer" is the hidden message; that's obvious. For uncertainty about it can keep you terrifically preoccupied for a long time. If only you knew what the truth really was! If there's nothing, well then, just live your life and don't get all hot and bothered about it, but just keep on breathing until you lay down your weary head, and then your mind will be at rest about everlasting rest.

And if there *is* something, then at least you can come to terms with it, then you know why you're doing it, and the certainty will give you a foundation and a handhold in this risky, embarrassing, burdensome life. "Make me more of a believer" is the message. "There are people who seem to know the furniture in heaven and the temperature in hell. I don't.

"Sometimes I hope that dead is dead; it seems to me that it's been nice enough. I'm so tired, I don't really feel very much like having to rise again. I think the Lord God won't be that eager to see me; I'll have to own up to things terribly. And I don't know if I'll want to see myself back, either. And sometimes I can get hopelessly sad at the thought that this is all there is, and that it'll never be all taken care of, that so much is left unfixed and un-understood. I wonder if this is all I really have to look forward to, and I secretly hope not, but how should *I* know?

"How must I number my days? Perhaps you know something more, and maybe you've got words for that great mystery."

★   ★   ★

Another stereotype that keeps coming up, especially for the priest, but sometimes also for the minister, is that of the Pope. "There comes the Pope," they say, or, "Are you bringing greetings from the Pope?" or, "Don't you think it's too bad that you can never be Pope?" or, "Holy Father, thou art come on foot; where's your sedan chair?" These associations are always connected with power and might.

Often the challenge has the overtone of "Show us your power." And there's anger, too: "You're useless; you can't get us down from the cross, you can't save us; you're impotent like the Pope and like the so-called Almighty God."

In all this there's a note of longing for someone who does have power, who needs to "speak but one word," a word with power, and we shall be healed. "Oh, that one star might twinkle above the misery, that there were one person stronger than our despondency and powerlessness, someone who could take over."

And through all of it there's also that note of longing that you yourself could be that person, that you might have power over yourself, that you could master yourself and at long last could be whom you want to be: a free, creative, luminous person.

Sometimes someone knelt down in front of you in the clinic and begged jeeringly for a blessing.

One day, fishing out at sea, they said, waving invitingly toward the surface of the water, "Well, preacher, go ahead, it's the chance of a lifetime!"

All kidding aside: how splendid it would be if a person came forward in the name of God before whom we could kneel down honestly, who would reach out and touch us and give us a blessing. Someone who, when the water is up to our chins, has the water under his feet, and who would prepare us a way to the other side.

★　★　★

A lot of them immediately begin talking about the church of the past. Their concern is not the actual situation, but the lost paradise. "We used to have High Mass; that was great," and they give you a colorful description, so that you can almost smell the atmosphere, a picture of I don't know how many priests at the altar, and how the choir could sing, and the bishop marching in and the organ and the flowers and the incense and all that—but it's all gone now, nothing is left of it. It's become cold and bare and barren in the church.

Protestants have fewer colors and odors to go back to, but even with them you get the disillusionment right under the surface: "I was baptized in the Ebenezer Church—they've torn it down now—people used to stand in line—you could hear Harry Vincent Coffrick then—wonderful speaker he was—and without a microphone, too—that man had a wonderful voice—just like, well, I don't know what—and all of it from memory, too—you could hear a pin drop—and when they started singing you'd think that the walls were going to come tumbling down, you really would."

You can see how much good it does people to bring that lovely past to life again by talking about it. What faith there was then! And suppose that by some miracle it was brought back to life?

With that question you often seem to stir up deeper sadness, because what you'd bring back to life would probably have no chance to survive. You've gotten older, and your soul is cold and bare and barren. You can't enter into that kingdom like a little child anymore. You've been through too much; you'd probably see right through it; it'd be an empty experience; and it could never really take you back. No, it's all in the past. "You can't go home again," says Thomas Wolfe. You can remain connected with the past only by living with the awareness that it's lost forever.

★ ★ ★

"You're not coming to hear my confession, are you?"

"Sorry, Chaplain, no sinners here."

"Jerry, there's the priest, better get ready to confess."

Just as I glance at my speedometer when I see a policeman, so does the appearance of a minister bring up thoughts of sin and guilt. Even before we've said a word, we have (according to many) called out, "Adam, where are you?" and people leap into the bushes or push others out into view. It seems as though people have a double attitude about all this. You want to talk about it, and you don't want to hear about it. You long for God who fathoms your heart, but you're mortally afraid, too. You gladly hear the psalm that begins "O Lord, Thou hast searched me and known me," and at the same time you don't want to let him know you.

Catholics speak with the same ambivalence about confession. On the one hand: "What an unbearable nuisance it was, good that they're not so stiff about making you do it anymore, such a spiritual launderette; sometimes you simply made up a story and then you were let off with this or that penance." And on the other hand: "It always did me a lot of good. What you never dared say to anyone else you could unload there, and you could breathe easy again, and you got your strength back—I don't understand how you priests could so easily let that powerful tool go and just use confessionals to store bass fiddles."

★ ★ ★

And there are also many who identify religion with morality and say, "I give everybody his due; I just try to live up to the Ten Commandments, and everybody should do that, just be good to your fellow man, that's what I always say, and that's what I do. I give to all the collections, no matter what church they're connected with. I'm quite broad-minded about that, they never come to me in vain—you can ask anybody. That's what faith is all about, living right, and if people only did that, it would be a paradise here, that's what I think."

They don't let themselves get in touch with other thoughts and feelings about what else religion might be; they've reduced faith to morality, and this pharasaic reduction lets them live in a faith that never tests their certainties and in which they can be secure for time and eternity. They don't want to expand their faith into an area which they're afraid they won't be able to master. They're very limited people, with boundaries, and they aren't broad-minded about that.

Faith Stories

They were sitting in a circle and telling each other their faith stories, and how they had ended up in our Westerkerk.

One said, "I fought with God very hard. For I lost my husband, and I held God responsible for that, and I just kept saying, But why? But why? and I got no answer at all, and I didn't want to hear anything more about God. Stick it in your ear, I thought. But it wouldn't let me alone—or He wouldn't let me alone; I don't know how I ought to say it. And one Sunday I walked into church here, and then the minister said, 'God doesn't take *away*. God takes us *home*. And that's quite different. God does not want pain and death.' And then that was such a relief to me that I could think that God doesn't stand over against me in my pain, but beside me. That's a great comfort for me. I found God again here."

★ ★ ★

Others told their stories, how—often after many wanderings of body and soul—they'd found a foothold here. And someone said, "What you just now said, about God and pain, that's how I experience it too. It touched me, what you said. There's a very important story in my life, and that's what I'll tell.

"I was born in this area, here in the Jordaan. I was baptized in this church, and I went to Sunday school here. I was still a little child when a little girl in the neighborhood died. A perfect darling she was, and everybody was terribly sad, of course. And I said, 'Don't cry, because the Lord Jesus will come soon and will raise Rosie from the dead.' They didn't want to believe that, but I believed it firmly. But after two days Jesus hadn't been there yet, and the day after that they plugged Rosie into the ground, and I was inconsolable. And furious. That evening my mother came to tuck me in, and I said, 'I'm not going to that Sunday school anymore, because all they do there is tell you fairy tales, and I'm not going to be hoodwinked any longer. I'm not going anymore.'

"My mother was a wise woman. She took me on her lap, and she said, 'Now you must listen to me carefully.' (I'll never forget how I sat there and what she said to me.) She said, 'Now just listen to me. Rosie had so much pain that the Lord Jesus said, Rose, come to me now, and you'll never have pain again.'

"Many a time my thoughts return to what my mother told me then. I'm forever grateful to her. And that's my story."

★   ★   ★

Two faith stories. From two people having opposing theologies, but who don't know that, and each of whom feels at home with the other's story.

That's curious. But if you think about it for a moment, it's not hard to understand. For what binds those two together is much stronger than what divides them. What both theologies have in common is their trust in God. The one trust in God is mediated by a minister who preached that God did *not* want this death, and the other by a mother who preached that God *did* want this death. But both preached God's goodness.

Good theology is important. But just as important is who says it. With an accurate theology you can mediate a crooked faith, and with a crooked theology you can mediate a straight faith. And about that I know another good story.

It's a story from my former supervisor Kwint, a gifted pastor in The Hague. And it's about a man who was set in high places, a despot who in the space of a single day, through a sudden sickness, was pulled down from his throne, put into the hospital, felled like an oak. A potentate without power, brought down below the level of his former subjects; a man who lived high on the hog in The Hague and then discovered to his horror that he was not God but a vulnerable mortal. And everybody in his vicinity had to suffer for it, so angry was the man. And our Lord's ground crew, the hospital chaplain who came to visit him, was heaped with abuse from him about that so-called almighty God of his. The pastor was denied the right to visit the room anymore.

The man's wife made contact with Kwint. Out of regard for the woman and also out of regard for the man who was seeing his kingdom shrink so, Kwint went to the hospital.

He opened the sickroom door. There lay the man, a wretched heap of humanity. "Then," as Kwint told the story years later, still shivering with the memory, "then I heard myself suddenly saying, 'I see that the Lord God's hit the bull's-eye this time.'

"Of course I should never have said that." Shocked, the man had pulled his head up from the pillow, looking for a word that would repel this cruel intruder with power, but he couldn't utter a word and fell back into the pillows like a wounded beast. And he wept. He wept bitterly. And Kwint went to him and stayed with him.

Poor theology.

Marvelous pastoral care.

Hospitable Church

(1)

The boy in prison was in a dilemma about whether he'd go to church on Christmas Eve or not. He longed to go, and at the same time resisted it just as much. "It's beautiful but also difficult to see Christmas," he said.

"What do you see when you see Christmas?" I asked.

"Then I see a family," he said.

The Hans Christian Andersen tale about the little match girl would have appealed to him: just as deprived and displaced and defenseless as he in a bitter-cold world, she lit in the night the matches she couldn't sell, and thus got a little heat and protection. She saw a stove burning in a cheerful room, and a roast goose on the table, stuffed with apples and prunes.

But the story of the little match girl ends well. In a vision she feels herself taken up by her grandmother in heaven, higher and yet higher, toward light and splendor, where there is no more hunger or cold. The next day people find her dead, but with a smile of happiness on her face.

The little girl is allowed to live inside her vision, but the boy has to return to a world where he can't see Christmas, but longs for it so.

★　★　★

In a few days people will once again go to church by the thousands to catch a glimpse of Christmas. In many churches they aren't very welcome. As the poet Paul van Ostayen puts it, a Teuton is a mammal that seeks out an evergreen tree at the end of December; and in many churches they don't trust animals like that, with their momentary religious belching, who then take their distance for another year. After all, they are nothing but pleasure-seekers, people think, who come for the atmosphere and get mad if they're not allowed to sing "Joy to the World." They rejoice when the Christ Child arrives but no longer take part when the child becomes a man and has something to say.

I've also gone through a period when those Christmas Eve

crowds irked me; in those dark days what helped me was that old joke about the man who went to church only on Christmas, but not every Christmas, because he didn't want to get into a rut.

And once in my old parish in North Holland at a Christmas Eve service, after a couple of announcements about the communicants' class and who would get the flowers, I came out with the following: "And now an announcement for those who are interested: the next Christmas service will be held next year at Christmas, at eleven o'clock in this church."

★ ★ ★

A people's church or an elite church: that's an old dilemma, and the tension between the two can also be found in the gospels. On the one hand you have the multitudes, the gathered flock, all one hundred of the sheep, the nations, and all those who labor and are heavy laden: the weirdest sorts of fish caught in the dragnet of the kingdom. And on the other hand it's stated that the way is strait, and the gate narrow, and one must obviously choose, because whoever is not for is against. If you want to escape from this dilemma and remove the tension between the two by taking one position or the other, you will do violence either to the hospitality of the church or to its radicality.

★ ★ ★

We need people who get concerned about a soupy sentimentalization of church and religion that mutilates the gospel and renders it innocuous.

But we also need people who get concerned about the beatification of radicality and who declare themselves for a hospitable church that neither blames nor screams, but preaches the Word without shortening or distorting, and always with kindness and trust, with an understanding of weakness and a sense of gradualness, both to haves and to have-nots, intellectuals and workers, progressives and conservatives—all deprived, displaced, and defenseless in a horribly cold, complicated world, like the little match girl—full of unfulfilled desires, searching for warmth and meaning.

A good church has particular appreciation and care for the "household of faith," but it won't refuse the identity card of Christian fellowship to those who show up irregularly or only at the high moments of life. A hospitable church extends jovial hospitality.

★ ★ ★

These are words from the bishop of Brugge. The name of that town means "bridges," and he is a true bridge builder. He pleads for a mild and warm church fellowship, hospitable to workers who've come to work at the first hour as well as to those who turn up only once a year at the eleventh hour. A church where you can find shelter, merciful and solid like a family.

(2)

"People are dying and are not happy."

It's painted on a wall somewhere in Amsterdam; I go by it every day.

Weird thought: some night a guy leaves his house somewhere in town with a ladder and a bucket of paint, climbs up a wall, screams out in big letters that people are dying and are unhappy, climbs down again, and goes back home, very sad and a bit happy at the same time.

I feel some sympathy with that man. I've had those words running around in my mind for years. They are words that Camus gives Caligula to say in the play of that name. I once had a part in that play. I've forgotten my own role, but not those words.

There's another sentence in that play that will always stay with me. The words are spoken by young Scipio. He hates Caligula, and he loves him. He has to choose for or against the emperor, but he can't do it. And with a divided and doubting heart he cries out, "As far as I'm concerned no one, no one will ever be right again."

You find the same sorrow, but tempered with fun and thus made bearable, in an unforgettable story by Sholom Aleichem, "Tevye the Dairyman." Somebody tells Tevye what he thinks about something. "You're right," says Tevye. Another man comes and says that his opinion is quite different. "You're right," says Tevye. "Listen to that," says Tevye's wife. "First you tell one man he's right, and then somebody comes along with the opposite opinion, and you tell him he's right!" "You know what?" says Tevye. "You're right."

I get so sick of people who are right. They're on my radio all days, unhindered by a drop of doubt, believing their beliefs; and if it has to do with something I don't know very much about, I'm usually in agreement with the last speaker.

But I also get that feeling in connection with things that I do know something about. The new hymnbook for the Dutch Protestant churches, for instance. Of course, "Silent Night" doesn't belong in it; by any reasonable standard it's a very weak hymn. And do we sing it on Christmas in the Westerkerk? Of course we do, because by any reasonable standard it's a lovely song, and I don't put the worship service together all by myself, and I love people who love that hymn, and, besides, it does me good to keep in touch with the person I once was.

People in whose houses I visit read *People* magazine, find pop religion deeply spiritual, and are deeply moved by the Andy Williams Christmas show. On the wall in their living room hangs a picture, painted on velvet, of a gypsy girl with a big bosom. On their way to Florida for a vacation, they sing songs out of the Mickey Mouse Hymnbook. These people say of the hymnbook (undeniably a product of a highly stylized emotional life) that its words and music give little voice to what runs deep within them. And in large numbers they illustrate that by tuning in to the Popular Hymn Hour for the Sick on the Evangelical Radio Station. And quite a number of them join creepy groups where tunes in 3/4 or 6/8 time are still favored. So those who, like me, are deeply grateful for the treasury of hymns in our hymnbook aren't the only ones who are right. Also right are the people who are just plain uneasy about our high-minded avoidance of a lot of folk religion.

★　★　★

We speak slightingly of "sociological Christians," and out of the necessity of declining numbers we make a virtue of increasing quality, but the French sociologist of religion Bonnet mockingly introduces the term *socio-cultural ministers*, challenging ministers to search their own hearts, because spirituality is always socio-culturally determined.

Bonnet reproaches priests that they're running around heedless of the pearls of great price you can find in folk religion. He doesn't call folk religion sacred—it, too, needs cleaning up and lifting up—but you must begin (a golden precept) where *people* are, and wherever that is, there you must pay careful attention to the riches and meaning of their faith. In fact, you must pay extra attention to it, because so little of it is expressed in words and logic.

Another argument, no less weighty, for listening to folk religion with respect and for not judging it on the grounds of superficial spirituality or buying it prematurely as worthless, is the conviction that the church itself, from the way it dealt with things in earlier years, is partly responsible for the very existence of a number of religious conceptions and practices.

God save us from "mature" Christians who shrink the gospel to its social relevance, who confuse maturity with a certain level of intellect and articulateness, and who shut out the voices of ordinary people and rob them of the vital supply lines of their faith.

God give us a little unity. After all, we are all people who are dying and who are looking for happiness. Aren't we?

Cemetery

"There's no field more fruitful than the field of the dead."

An elder in my village in North Holland used to say that whenever I complained about people who never set foot in the church but nevertheless always came to hire you for a funeral.

I said that if he saw as few seeds germinate in the field behind his farmhouse as I did in the cemetery behind the church, he might as well hang his overalls on a willow tree. But then *he* said in his own way what the poet A. Roland Holst said in these lines:

I'll never see the ears of corn
Nor bind the sheaves so full
But let me trust that harvest comes
For which I serve.

And I took heart again.

Uneasy about taking part in a hypocritical ceremony, I tried just once to refuse to perform a funeral. In those days I was still in search of my own identity and just couldn't let people walk all over me. But the widow beseeched me not to let her husband be put into the ground like a dog, and then we agreed that I'd say something at their home and keep quiet at the graveside. I'd just read a book full of churchy babble about the messianic community which buries one of its members with Easter hymns and the Lord's Prayer, and I was asking myself as a matter of principle why you'd suddenly start saying prayers in the graveyard with people who never say any prayers in church.

So: no Lord's Prayer. It was, all in all, a barren affair, standing there like that, and I by the grave being as silent as the grave. The undertaker made a gesture that it was time to leave, and I made an encouraging sign to the widow. And then she said—I shall never forget that beseeching tone, nor the sidelong glance she threw at me through her tears—"Please, Reverend, one tiny Lord's Prayer." Gently but firmly, I refused. The servant of the Lord who let himself be mocked at did not want to be mocked at.

Now I live a long way from farm fields or cemeteries. I live in Amsterdam, that big city where people's houses stand on pilings but their faith is sagging. But here and there you will still find fragments. And at times of strong emotions—at births, marriages, and deaths—you see people trying to piece the fragments together.

Not long ago another woman called me up. Would I do a funeral? I would. She wanted a really nice funeral and could I help? I could. "How did you happen to choose me?" I asked. "I found you in the yellow pages," she said.

Well, whether they get my name from the Lord himself or whether I get a job out of the yellow pages, that's the least of my concerns! I used to get myself all annoyed about the poverty of many people's faith and the draggy hymns they like to sing. It wasn't without a certain haughtiness that I talked about "religion." I didn't want any part of that. I'd learned my Barth; religion, according to Barth, is "unfaith." But since my conversion, I've been busy learning no longer to be misled by the often small power of expression of people and to listen very thoughtfully to the beauty in that "poverty" and not to "quench the smoking flax." Religion can be opium but it can also be oxygen, and in any case you have to begin by taking people as they are, in the trust that a longing for faith can grow out of religious needs, and hope out of wishes.

Heavens, maybe that elder was right after all with his fantasies about what might possibly grow in the fruitful field of the dead.

Mourning

Some weeks ago I was called on for a consultation by a family doctor. He'd been asked to conduct a funeral.

"If I understand it right," I said, "the medicine man again has to become a priest, as well?"

"You've got it," he said, "if the priests leave such a gap in the market."

A father and mother had lost their child and were at their wits' end. They'd considered seeking solace in the rites of the church, with its treasury of hymns and prayers that give voice to grief, cast light on the dignity of the dead, and honor their living and dying. But in fact they found it more honest not to do that. It was no longer a part of their lives, and they wanted to be consistent. But they really didn't know how to get through that day; they didn't want to bury their beloved child just like that, without a word, without a gesture. Couldn't the doctor help? And the doctor asked me if *I* could.

I once got a similar question from a psychologist. In the nursing home where he worked, people would spirit away the dead, take them out on the sly. Nothing was said about the deceased and about death, and so the psychologist had discovered a lot of stopped-up grief. "Do you have any experience with group work for grieving people?" he asked.

"For centuries," I said.

And I proposed that from then on we should make a circuit of the pavilion with the body, with the priest leading, swinging first his tassels and then his censer, then I would come next with a heavy Bible, followed by the sisters, veiled in black and giving their tears free rein. The psychologist agreed with me that we'd spruce the whole place up considerably that way. Well, we were being a bit sarcastic.

★ ★ ★

Far more seriously, I thought long into the night with the doctor about the psychological health issues involved in funerals, and how you could best help people to express and bear their grief. Around them are gathered other mortals who are also shocked to death; how can you bring all these people into a unity around this one dead human being? We did our best to think of new rites to give form to sorrow.

I did it with all the more energy because I was still immensely upset by the secularized funeral of a non-religious friend whose death caused me great grief. His boss and one of his colleagues wearied us with ineffable baloney; it made you cry, but exactly *not* the kind of tears you needed to shed just then. And when after that short and creepy "unceremony" we sat down to a funeral lunch, I regretted not having stepped forward to remember this man with a few words about his life, so rich and so poor, about the belief from which he'd had to free himself, and the unbelief with which he'd tried to make it in this life. Moreover, I think, I ought to have told a couple of jokes, for he was a gifted fool and he'd have been grateful for a last rite with some humor in it.

★ ★ ★

A few days after that dismal experience I attended a requiem Mass. The priest did just about nothing right: his sermon was very superficial; from the text of the mortuary card, one would judge that he was not hindered by any spiritual baggage; the choir sang wretchedly. Yet what a lovely service it was. Impressive, and I really mean that. Indestructible bits from the Bible, songs, prayers, and gestures expressed our sorrow and our loneliness—and our anger, gratitude, guilt, and affection, too. Death was plainly called death. Six candles stood around the coffin. "Two at my head, two at my feet, and two to light my way to paradise," I meditated, recalling that old children's bedtime prayer that begins,

> When at night I go to sleep,
> Fourteen angels watch do keep . . .

And in the midst of music that was being sung from generation to generation, you could shed some tears. No, it was really a lovely service; I was glad I'd gone; it did me a world of good.

From Johan Huizinga we learn that rituals give rhythm to sorrow. Ph. Rümke argues for a revival of the cult of death; he called it a task of the deepest importance for mental health care. And though you can't change a cultural pattern overnight, it's nonetheless certainly good to have a sleepless night over it now and then.

Hoping and Wishing

The boy had told me about his future, full of hope. After much sorrow, life was smiling at him again. He'd received an inheritance—a lot of money and a small house far from here in a distant land in a lonely spot in a huge forest. As soon as he got out of prison, he would look for a wife and find one and then go live there. They'd have children and would live long and happily.

It was a joyful story, and he told it so winningly, entered into it so fully. But there was something that held me back from going along with him. *Don't get suckered*, said a voice in me, catching on that the whole story was aimed at entrapping that person in me who loves stories of peace and resurrection so much. There *was* absolutely no inheritance, no money, no house far from this scene of his misfortune, in a great forest in a lonely spot, far from people who don't love you, whom you can't trust, and who don't trust you.

It was his song of longing: a woman with children around her skirts, who waits for you in the doorway and says, "Come on in, dear, you must be tired. I've been standing here waiting for you. It's cold out there, but the coffee's ready."

★   ★   ★

If a child has a nightmare, then you wake the child up, hold it close, give it something to drink. That does the child good; you wake it out of its anxiety of death into life.

When that boy told me his lovely dream, I didn't know what to do. Who am I to wake him out of his dream of peace and take him back into the nightmare of his reality? If that dream was keeping him alive, should I then . . . ? But I couldn't hide my confusion very well. We looked at each other.

"You've told me your dream," I had to say.

He talked about being abandoned. "That happened long, long ago," he said, but with so much emphasis that I had to ask for clarification.

"It all happened in an earlier life," he said.

"It all began in an earlier life?" I asked.

"Yeah," he said.

"And maybe you have the feeling that it won't stop until another life?"

"Yeah."

★   ★   ★

The Easter story offers many people a handhold comparable to the young man's dream of a land far from here where life is good: the Father stands in the doorway waiting for his Son and says, "Come on in, boy, how tired and worn out you must be! I've been standing here watching to see if you'd come. Let's sit down and eat." Then the Father gives orders to his servants to kill the fatted calf, for "My Son here was dead and is alive again, the night is at an end, the evil dream has passed."

Stand up, an unexpected day
God's day has dawned.

The morning is full of new sounds,
Throw off your evil dreams.

I've learned to make a distinction between dreams based on wishes and dreams based on hope.

Easter can be a dream in the service of wishes. You stuff an empty present with pious wish-fulfillment fantasies, and then you enter into that vision, and you try to bring others to that same belief, for what many people believe is more probable than what you believe all by yourself.

Easter can also be a dream filled with hope that gives life. Then wish-fulfillment dreams are seen as evil dreams that must be thrown off, because they cripple us instead of stimulating us toward growth and change, and because they block the future instead of making it accessible.

★ ★ ★

People have to help one another to hope, help each other to dream so that you don't have to flee from a sad past or a paltry present to a land far away. The road to life lies straight before us, when we believe that the pain of looking at the past and the present can be borne, and that we descend into hell expecting to ascend into heaven.

Morning Blessing

The sexton told me a woman had called to ask if I would come to her house the following week to bring the morning blessing on the occasion of her seventieth birthday.

I liked the idea immediately.

"What's a morning blessing, really?" asked the sexton.

"That I don't know," I said, "but I'm definitely going to find out, and I'm certainly going to take one to her."

Later that day the old black woman told me how, on her sixty-fifth birthday, while she was still living in Paramaribo, the minister had come to bring her the morning blessing. She'd like to have it just the same now—prayers, Bible readings, preaching, psalms, and hymns. At eleven in the morning at her home. With her seven sons and three daughters, of whom some had come all the way from Surinam especially.

She lives in the Kinker neighborhood.

As I walk there I feel for a moment like that little ragamuffin who toted wood out of abandoned houses during the "Hunger Winter" of World War II right by the barbed wire where the minefield began.

★ ★ ★

We sang a hymn, and I read Psalm 23. "The Lord is my shepherd, I shall not want," and that was especially underlined by the children who at that moment came in late with impressive loads of food and drink. The cup was obviously running over, and I had to think of that wonderful Easter sermon by Saint John Chrysostom: "Be joyful this day! The table is bending under the weight of the food, and all may come and enjoy. The fatted calf is ready, no one need go away empty. All of you, eat your fill at this flood of God's goodness."

★ ★ ★

It was good, yes, very good, and so the minister can say a final amen, but they had no need of such an amen and went right on; for God's mercy endureth forever and a person may at least take a bit of that eternity so as to be able to praise the Lord.

The songs we sang! Dutch, English, and Surinamese songs, solos, rounds, refrains—and if the song was beautiful and made us feel good, it was repeated twice, three times, four times, because the experience grows when you repeat the praises "to all eternity." We sang "Count Your Blessings" and "Lo! He Comes" and many songs that must have been born in slavery, in which oppressed people gather up all the courage of their faith and never become weary of reminding one another that the Lord Jesus loves us, that he does not leave us alone in the valley of the shadow of death, and that wherever we go he goes with us.

How deeply I identified myself with these people and their history I realized when at a particular moment I fantasized that an overseer came in with his whip and *we* just went right on singing.

★   ★   ★

We alternated religious and secular repertoire with great mental agility:

Under Akke Franke's bridge
There oak wood is sold.
But that wood, it will not burn,
And you will stay cold.
What a lot of grief!
Don't buy wood from Akke Franke,
For he is a thief!

We sang that, and one of the sons took the role of Akke Franke, and sprang up more and more angrily each time he was identified as a thief.

His jumping up and down had made it difficult for him to see the songbook, but nonetheless he found what he was looking for, and off we went with the old psalm: "Behold, how good, how lovely it is, when sons of the same house dwell together as brothers."

★   ★   ★

The daughters went to stand around their mother and sang God's blessing to her. The sons went to stand around their mother and sang that even if you have all the world's gold and have no mother, you're as poor as a churchmouse. Fortunately, they had both gold and mother, and we drank some champagne.

Several of them danced with the birthday girl a bit and sang a song of birthday wishes to her: "I came to congratulate you, I didn't come for all the goodies, but they sure are good!"

We said cordial good-byes to one another. I promised to return soon. I know they won't come to see me. We don't dance in church. We do sing about sadness and joy, but in such a highly stylized way that they can scarcely feel it, and we sing almost nothing in 3/4 time, and we always sing only one song, and then you have to listen again for a long, long time. And among us only those with a couple of the proper graduate degrees are allowed to talk about the Carpenter, and that's quite obvious, too!

I was thinking of all that as I walked home. Back to worrying again, I must admit.

But it occurred to me that the shabby neighborhood looked a lot different from the way it looked before.

Calling

"Father and Mother Stolk, by what name do you wish your child to be called, now and in the life eternal?"

"Anna Elisabeth," said her parents at the baptismal service.

I always find that a wonderful moment, but of course you never know if anyone else experiences it that way.

"Why do people get names?" I asked the children in church, who always crowd as far forward as they can at baptisms.

"Well," said a little girl, "then they can call you."

I asked who "they" were.

"Your mom and dad," said one.

"Your friend," said another.

"God," said a boy.

You always have to be careful with answers like that. They can come straight from the heart, but also from a kind of God-talk triggered off by opportunism. Once I had a child in church who always cried out "The Holy Ghost!" before I'd had a chance to ask anything.

"God," said the boy. I saw that he meant it, and the kid next to him thought it was a good answer, but another child didn't. A God who calls? He could scarcely imagine that.

★   ★   ★

It's the same with adults: some feel called; others know nothing of calling.

"Chaplain, do you have a call?"

They often asked me that in prison. For years I'd had an evasive answer for that in my repertory, until I discovered to my shame that I'd never heard what these people really were asking. Of course, they didn't want to know about me so much as they wanted to know something about themselves. "Do you have experience with a God who calls? If so, please tell us about that, because we've never heard God calling—or does that make any sense, that some people hear something from God and others don't?"

Yes, calling: how does it work?

It never comes falling out of heaven just like that. Calling is always mediated, transmitted through people, a book, an event. There's no voice direct from above; there's a voice from within, the experience of a burning desire for a particular task, and the power to perform it. It comes entirely from within, but at the same time it overpowers you and you feel as though you have to pray and say "Gracious God," or something like that.

With others you can talk about such an experience only with difficulty. You're vulnerable. But sometimes it works out right, as it did recently on a weekend with a church membership class. They were sitting in a big circle taking turns telling one another their life stories and the adventures of their faith. That was unusually beautiful; twenty-four splendid stories. One girl said that she didn't have so much to tell as the others. She'd grown up in a church family, but that wasn't the only reason she wanted to be confirmed; it was really something having to do with herself, she said. "Do you want to hear more about it?"

Yes, we wanted to hear more. We wanted to know how that had happened, that it was something having to do with herself.

She hesitated. "Maybe it's really quite silly," she said. Then she told how in the hospital (where she was a student nurse) the head nurse had approached her and had said, "Mr. Van Asselt asked for you tonight; he'd really like to talk with you." "And then, I don't know if the head nurse noticed, but a tremendous feeling of happiness rushed through me. I don't know how to say it, but I got tears in my eyes, and then I quickly moved on."

She looked around rather shyly, obviously afraid that someone would invite her to say more, not only about Mr. Van Asselt but also about God. But everyone had understood perfectly well that she had told about a call, how the bramble bush of her life had been set afire, that her name had been called, and that her floor in the hospital had become holy ground.

"What a beautiful story that was," I said later that evening when we were still sitting together for a while.

"Really?" she said, and immediately plucked up courage for the sequel. Mr. Van Asselt had gone home, but it hadn't gone well, and after a week or so he'd come back. And the first thing he asked was whether she was still on the unit.

Such a story tells you something more about calling. Not simply that it doesn't come falling out of heaven, but also that it's never a one-shot occurrence but has to grow and ripen. I think that the ancient writer meant something like that with the story about the young Samuel, who heard his name called three times and gradually caught on that God was really dealing with him.

★　★　★

A tremendous feeling of happiness overcomes you when you've found your calling. And despair can overtake you if, for the love of God, you don't know why you're here. In Amsterdam there are thousands of people like that walking around. Nobody calls them; they're nameless. They really don't know how they're to make their mark on history, and with wild abandon they paint their names and the names of the idols they identify with—the chosen who have made it—on walls and fences, buses and bridges, streetcars and sidewalks. They get a kick out of that, out of this work of their hands with spray cans and marker pens and paintbrushes on all kinds of movable and immovable objects. For a moment they can live in the illusion of really being somebody, even perhaps one of the elect. But in their hearts they really know better. *"Trix is ook nix"* (Queen Beatrix is nobody either), it says here and there in big letters. That "either" strikes me particularly. It slops back upon the painter himself. He reveals to us that he is nobody and comforts himself with the thought that someone he sees as privileged is nobody either.

Meanwhile, don't think that I despise these painters and

chalkers. I don't do such splashing myself because I have something else to do, but that's just the point; that's why you have to be sympathetic to the fate of so many who really *don't* have something else to do—people without a calling, often without a job at all, who have to kill time because they can't live it. *"Geen woning, geen kroning,"* they scribble—no housing, no coronation. They scream for a place to live, but the real pain lies somewhat deeper: they're walking around at loose ends. They are the Spiritually Homeless.

★   ★   ★

Besides, it isn't true that only fools and asses write their names on walls and glasses. Who doesn't want to see or hear his name? Anna Elisabeth doesn't know her Christian name yet. But soon enough she'll surely be fascinated by it, and she'll try to find out what kind of life goes with it. And her father and mother will see her practicing a characteristic signature hour after hour, and one day they'll find a scrap of paper in her room, her first calling card: Anna Elisabeth Stolk, Keizersgracht 249, Amsterdam, North Holland, the Netherlands, Europe, the World, the Universe. And that's how a little Anna creates for herself a place to live.

And I still remember quite well what ran through me as a little boy, when we sang:

His eye is on the sparrow,
And I know He watches me.

As a matter of fact, I believe I still believe that.

Questions

Still tired from Sunday, I was already debating with myself on Monday about next week's sermon. I have a wonderful profession, but sometimes it's a lousy job.

I hesitated whether to deal with "Questions," based on that story Jesus told about the widow who was out in the cold but kept pestering the judge with her questions until she got what she wanted, or with the calling of Nathanael, who heard from Jesus that he would see the old dream of Jacob about a ladder to heaven fulfilled. I still hadn't decided when the young woman who'd asked to see me arrived.

★ ★ ★

"I don't know very well how to begin. I've got so many questions. At first I thought I could manage. But I haven't got very far. It's been on my mind for several months. I've got some things clear, but not others; I can't shake them, and that's what I want to talk about. A few months ago I lost a very good friend. That's sad in itself, and I'd never had that happen before. But she didn't just die. She committed suicide.

"That really laid me low. Now it's going a little better, but the grief is still there. And the bitter feeling that happiness is so unevenly distributed. I've also become afraid. For my happiness can go ker-flooey too. People are vulnerable; I've caught on to that. It doesn't take much to throw you completely off balance.

"And I feel guilty, too. Because I'm alive. And that's not the only reason. My friend wanted to talk to me about her desire to escape this life. But I didn't want to. Couldn't. Really, it was only afterward that I noticed that I'd carefully avoided that painful subject and ducked whenever she brought it up. For her sake, I thought then, but now I know it was for my own. And so I managed to make her even lonelier than she already was. I'm shocked at myself. You want to be able to do so much, and you can do so little.

"We talked for hours and I tried so hard to give her some courage, some hope, some warmth. But it didn't work. Her death makes me angry, too. Yes, at first you don't dare admit that—it's a sort of forbidden feeling—but I'll be honest with you, I'm really awfully angry at her. I know that that's not entirely right, but that's how I feel anyhow. For she didn't just do something to herself, she did something to me, too! My whole life's been changed by it. I'll never again be who I was."

★ ★ ★

The young woman told me about one of their last meetings, a walk in the hospital garden. In that garden was a stairway, a rather steep one up to a terrace. While they were climbing, her friend had said that on these stairs she always thought of Jacob's dream, the dream of a ladder to heaven.

"Do you think your friend's in heaven now?" I asked.

"I don't know. Everything nailed down is coming loose, even my faith. Too many questions. I don't understand God. Before this happened, I always believed. And I never knew any better than to think it would always last. In any case, I'm through with my earlier faith. My faith is never again going to be what it was, either.

"A friend of mine says that I ought to stop brooding. He thinks I should say good-bye to God, and then things would go better. He says I'll find 'it' in oriental meditation. That's where I'll get myself back, he says, that's where I'll find the peace I'm looking for. But I know I mustn't get into that. I have to stick with God, I think. I don't know exactly how to say it. Even if it's something from the past, it's very dear to me. My experiences from the past aren't nothing. And there is the faith of those I love. That's where I've got to look for it, even though I don't know where to start looking."

★   ★   ★

Her story moved me. It may well be a lousy job, but sometimes it's a wonderful profession! As she saw it, she had confided her unbelief to me; but as I saw it, hers was a tale of faith. For what is believing? Knowing the right answers? Or daring to live with the right questions?

★   ★   ★

We divide people up in this world mostly according to skin color or race or religious preference. But there is a division that runs much deeper: people who still ask questions and people who've given up asking. And the only thing I could say to that young woman was: please keep on with your questions. You ask so bravely. In God's name, try to bear the pain and keep your questions open. Faith that can't face questions doesn't go anywhere. If believing is anything at all, if it isn't just poppycock, if God really stands behind it, then he can stand our questions. If you don't ask questions any longer, you no longer grow. Children keep asking questions; it's part of growing up: "What keeps the stars in the sky? Where does the snow come from? Does the rain have a father? Where was I when there wasn't anything yet?" If you don't ask any longer, you grow dense.

Go on with your questions. Just like Job. He never stopped. His wife advised him to seek his salvation somewhere else; she thought he'd get rid of his misery if he got rid of God. She thought Job ought to say good-bye to God, and then things would go better. But Job couldn't say good-bye to God; his earlier experiences were too dear to him. And he'd rather go down in his own darkness than let himself be put off with cheap answers.

★ ★ ★

Go on with your questions. Just like that widow. Bereft and downcast in a cold world, she pestered that judge half to death with her questions. And she kept on. And Jesus called that questioning *faith*. By asking questions we remain in touch with the wellsprings of life. And we remain receptive to God's questions. That's how the story of Job ends, with God's questions to Job: "What keeps the stars in the sky? Where does the snow come from? Does the rain have a father? Where were you when there wasn't anything yet?"

And it's with a question that Jesus ends his story about the widow: "When the Son of man comes, will he find faith upon the earth?"

Will there be questioners like that woman?

Looking

Looking is an art. Our eyes make selections, choose what they want to see. To the question, Does smoking cause cancer? most non-smokers say yes, and most smokers say no. It's all in how you look at it.

Our receiving apparatus not only chooses but modifies. Two people who look at the same thing often see it quite differently. How those views can differ is visible in the old joke about the shoe manufacturer who commissioned two pieces of market research in Central Africa. After a while he received two telegrams. The first telegram: NO CHANCES STOP NOBODY HERE WEARS SHOES. Second telegram: FANTASTIC POSSIBILITIES STOP NOBODY HERE WEARS SHOES.

Our eyes choose and then modify reality. In itself that's not troubling; the question is merely whether reality is accurately represented, whether our eyes "look rightly."

★ ★ ★

An old Jewish proverb says, "A righteous man cares for his beast."

An unrighteous person says, "An animal is just an animal, and I am I, and I'm the king." Such a person never looks at anything but himself. He is not receptive to the other who comes to him in the animal. The unrighteous person is dense, can't look.

There is a tale that tells how Jesus tries to teach those of little faith the art of looking, to make them receptive to the birds of the air and the lilies of the field. Look, says Jesus, they help you with your faith because they awaken wonder and testify to God's fatherly care.

The unrighteous person does not see it. He's a tourist munching french fries alongside his "wheels," who dares not wander into the woods and would rather stay where he can always hear the Top 40. For in nature he will always hear his own heart beating, will always hear himself breathing. He'll be confronted with himself and his finitude. It's difficult for him to bear the silence, and prayer no longer comes out right. He dares not enter *that* forest either; he'll get lost. Along the shores where there's deep water he becomes aware of his own superficiality, and he runs back to his four-door station wagon. He doesn't dare "wander lonely as a cloud . . . beneath the trees," and since he doesn't love "all things both great and small," he can't pray properly either.

The righteous person knows the value of his animals, keeps company with them like Noah in the ark.

"But the inward parts of the godless are cruel." So runs the second half of that proverb. The unrighteous man has covered himself with armor; walks with blinders on; cannot observe well; no longer knows wonder; no longer admits any religious questions; closes himself off from the other; closes himself off, too, from his own deep feelings; comes, you might say, no further than his own edges. Look at the animals, how they are destroyed, mishandled, and worn out, how creation sighs and groans in its depths, how mother earth is mistreated. Evil!

★ ★ ★

This week we commemorate Saint Francis, that wonderful boarder at the Lord's table, who dealt so nobly with animals, regarded Brother Sun and Sister Water with such respect and was grateful for Brother Wind and Mother Earth, who carries us and supplies us with fruits and flowers and herbs. Nature: Saint Francis looks at her with awe and listens to what she has to say. It is godless not to give nature that attention.

★ ★ ★

There is a village in our country where before Sunday, the holy day, the farmer takes the rooster out of the henhouse. It is very simple to ridicule that man; he probably has very distorted thoughts about sexuality and strange ideas about hallowing the sabbath. But at least he still has some ideas about it, and for me there is something moving about that scene: peace on the farm, it's the sabbath, and you shall not work, neither you nor your manservant nor your ox nor your ass. Refresh yourself; take a deep breath; look at the lilies and the birds; sing to the Creator a song of praise; and forget not, O man, how you, together with the animals, are created for the promise.

Is that farmer a fool?

God give us more such fools, with their beautiful pantomimes of salvation.

A fool like Saint Francis. Once he saw a worm lying on the road. He bowed, picked the worm up, and laid it in the grass by the road. And he told his friends how the Lord Jesus had compared himself to a worm when, on the cross, he made an ancient psalm of complaint his own because those words had to do with his own terrible experience: a worm am I and no man.

A fool like Albert Schweitzer. Once he was in Middelburg to give an organ concert. After dinner he was walking with his hostess through the garden of the house where he was to spend the night. A spider crept across the garden path, and the lady stepped on the spider and crushed it.

Schweitzer drew back and said, "Do you know how to make those?"

Born of God

Among the children that I had the privilege of baptizing on Sunday there was, besides a Surinamese child and a Dutch child, a Korean child, Kyung Kim. "In Christ there is no East or West, in him no South nor North," we sang, and in the meantime we got direct evidence of the rich differences in color that our Creator has on his palette.

For a few weeks now we have been meditating in our church on the old tales in the book of Samuel. Last Sunday we came to the story about Saul and Jonathan, and that was very fitting, as you'll see. Saul is conducting a war against the Philistines. But through a ruse concocted by his son, the battle is really won before it is under way. In an unguarded moment Saul has sworn that whoever takes a morsel of food before evening is accursed—but Jonathan has already eaten before he hears of his father's edict. That evening Saul, uncertain whether to pursue the fleeing enemy, has a priest inquire of God. But God is silent. Why? Who is the guilty one causing God's silence? "Even if it were my own son," cries Saul, "he shall surely die."

Why is he thinking of his own son Jonathan at this very moment? Is that accidental? Or is Saul betraying what lurks in a hidden corner of his soul?

I think it's the latter. Trapped by anxiety and ego-centered thinking, he begrudges his son the sympathy of the people. "Even if it were my own son," he cries out in phony righteousness, but meanwhile we see behind these royal words into a not-so-royal heart where jealousy reigns. A rich future for your children can be a wellspring of joy, but also an obsession. Saul was not the first and would not be the last: a person capable of offering his child upon the altar of his own prestige and ambition.

★ ★ ★

The story was very appropriate to tell at Kyung Kim's baptism. His father died in a far-off land, and his mother could no longer care for him. Only if she entrusted him to someone else would he have a future. And so it was mother love that made her part with him.

She had given Kyung a plant to take with him as a little greeting for his new mother. Somewhere on the way, Kyung forgot it, but the moving thought did come along with him as a costly gift.

Now the painful question is put to Kyung's new parents over and over again whether they think they can love him just as much as if he were their own child.

Why do people ask that? Or, if you don't actually ask it but think it, why do you think it? Just because of the uncertainty about the consequences of transplanting such a "tender shoot" out of a completely different culture into our own? I think it's more than that.

Do we love our children just because we have borne them?

It's very possible. In the prison where I worked, I've seen splendid examples of that. "Chaplain, the newspapers may say that he's a beast, but he's my son!" But I've also seen the most shocking examples of the opposite attitude. Who doesn't know the strife and bitterness of parents whose children have gone entirely different ways? How many parents feel rejected, betrayed: "My own flesh and blood . . . and now this!" How many lost sons and daughters are there with lost fathers and mothers?

I suspect that it's the deeply hidden fear of losing your own flesh and blood that makes people accentuate the lack of a blood connection in the case of an adoption: "Blood is thicker than water," they say. But it sounds like an incantation.

★ ★ ★

For that reason I felt, as I baptized Kyung Kim, that it was more meaningful than ever to ask the parents whether they solemnly promised to be faithful to their child, bearing in mind that he is born of God.

A question of fatherhood, then.

The parents made their vows in the same place where the stories of Jesus and his mother are told again and again: about the tenderness of their blood relationship, but also about its relativity. Love for his mother was of great importance to Jesus, but not of ultimate importance. "Blessed is the womb that bore you," cried a voice from the crowd, but Jesus put a different blessing up against that one. "Blessed are they who hear the word of God and do it."

Of his tender closeness to Mary and the unmistakable distance, too, that moving scene at the end of his life bears witness, when from the cross he says to his mother, "Woman, behold your son." And he gave his dear friend John a future with the words, "Behold your mother."

Gerard

I hadn't seen Gerard in years. He was still at the beginning of his life when I came to know him. A bashful boy. In youth camp he kept to himself and always walked behind the others in solitude, and you never knew which was better—trying to haul him along or leaving him alone. You never quite knew what to say to him.

And now we were meeting again. After fifteen years. In the hospital on Prince's Canal. Each of us knowing that now he was coming to the end of his life. So soon. And once again I was confused and didn't know what to say. Still it was a special visit, in any event for me. For when I walked outside, back into the land of the living, I thought, *Now he is ahead of us all.*

Exactly where he got it I don't know, but this perennial nursling lay dying like a man, brave, truly master of the sad situation, with a touching concern for others, especially for his parents and the friend he shared his life with, who cared for him equally touchingly. I thought, *Now he is ahead of us all.*

★ ★ ★

Others had that thought, too. When he had died, I asked his parents if there was a particular Bible story that had special meaning for them in these days. Yes, said his father, I keep thinking of that story of Paul taking leave of those dear to him because he was going to make a long journey. They all knew that they would never see each other again. So with tears they took leave of each other forever. But somehow Paul was master of this terrible situation; he knew that death awaited him yonder, and yet he was at peace with it, radiated power, and that power energized those who remained behind.

★ ★ ★

"How did you know I was here?" asked Gerard.

"Your mother telephoned."

He smiled. "Yes, she's always on the go with faith." And a moment later, "She's so uptight."

"Rightly so?"

"Yeah. I think I'm dying," said Gerard. "And I just have one hope: that they'll help me out of my pain when the time comes."

I fell silent. Was all further hope gone? I didn't dare speak. I'm from the church. Always on the go with faith and often too cheap and too smooth—and the silent ones like Gerard hear that very well. He also had a sharp antenna out for honesty and phoniness. And there's more to it than that: the church has often said awful things to people like Gerard. So I said nothing. Besides, I'm not dying yet. I'm letting him go ahead.

★ ★ ★

"Death is a black hole," said Gerard after a while. I had the feeling that he was testing me to see if I would set the door to heaven ajar a little. But he was more at peace now. "Maybe somebody has a purpose for all this," he said.

I asked him if he wasn't furious with that "somebody" and said that it surprised me that he could speak of that "somebody" with some trust.

"Maybe the anger's still to come," said Gerard, and after that he maintained that he believed God had a hidden meaning for this. Was that Gerard's way of keeping himself going? It was all right with me. In such situations you have to try not to fall apart, and so you sometimes have to resort to certain strategies.

Then Gerard said softly, "And maybe it'll mean something for people." Gratefully he recalled the letters which told him the things people ordinarily have so much difficulty saying: that he'd meant so much to them. "I had never realized that," said Gerard, and he cried.

★ ★ ★

A couple of weeks later he died, yet rather unexpectedly. Only the most intimate people in his life were with him at the end. His mother asked if she shouldn't warn me, but Gerard said that wasn't necessary. His mother said she thought that I had to be told, but Gerard said it really wasn't necessary. His mother said that she could imagine that in that case I'd have difficulty doing the funeral, but Gerard said I'd understand perfectly well. His mother asked what to do if I refused to conduct the funeral. "Then *you* just say the Lord's Prayer," said Gerard.

I think that's great, not to let the church get in the way of Our Father.

★ ★ ★

At the funeral I tried to find an answer to the question whether this life was now complete. A tough question, and it wasn't Gerard's style to sell onions and call them lemons.

Of course this life was not complete. He was still so young. We would have wished so much more for him. There was so much waiting to unfold that needed more thinking and ripening. He was a guy with so much depth that his faith would surely have deepened.

And still, just raising the question was a way of answering it positively. Gerard did not die; he gave up the ghost. "I am a child of God," he said to his parents. "He made me." In that basic trust communicated to him in a home that really was a home, through years that were often difficult, to that godawful, bitter, but beautiful end, he left us.

★　★　★

Sunday we celebrated All Saints' Day; we remembered our dead and named their names. Gerard was one of them. He always walked behind. Now he is ahead of us. One of the saints who from their labors rest. We sang about that.

The Old Wester Tower

For anyone who wants to sing some good old-fashioned songs, the Prince's Canal in Amsterdam is the place on a Sunday: in the morning the Wester Church, where we sing songs of praise wholeheartedly, and in the afternoon, across the canal, in the café called De Twee Zwaantjes, almost opposite the Anne Frank house, where a crew just as motley as the one in the church is bawling out the flowery repertoire of that area called the Jordaan.

You'll be glad you went.

They're songs of praise in both places and at both times hymns that celebrate creation and heaven, and also the Jordaan and the Westertoren, the great tower by our church.

In church we sing about the finger of God, "tow'ring o'er the wrecks of time," indicating that both time and eternity are of heaven. You'll feel like a different person.

And in the tavern we praise the old Wester Tower, the pearl of the Jordaan.

> Though cowhides are your foundations
> Though your top is made of wood,
> Still your bronze bells' exclamations
> Always make me feel so good.
> Then I see you made of gold,
> Standing proudly like a king
> In the sunshine as of old:
> Bring us new life, bells, and ring!

The café De Twee Zwaantjes (which means The Two Little Swans) is located near the bridge to the Lily Canal. Out its windows you can see the Wester. It was from just about this spot that Rembrandt sketched the tower.

The church and the tavern lie close by each other, and I'm more and more inclined to think that our songs don't lie so far from each other, either, although you might think so at the first hearing.

★   ★   ★

It was a Jordaner, a resident of the Jordaan area, who put this idea into my head. He was sitting with a group of fifteen people in my study as they told each other their personal and religious histories.

At a particular moment I asked the man if he would tell his story. He'd already seen the thunderheads gathering and was obviously not very comfortable. "I'm just an ordinary guy," he said. "I can't say things as nicely as those other folks. I come from here in the neighborhood, and if I go to church I go here. I think it's nice here, and I dunno what else t'say about it." He looked at me rather helplessly.

"Could you tell us a bit about what you think of when you walk across the Rose Canal on a Sunday morning?" I tried.

"Oh, sure, I can do that," he said. I knew he was happy with the question, because he immediately slid forward to the edge of his chair. "Then I see that tower. That's always so beautiful, that tower, so high in the air, really high." He looked around the circle for a moment, as if to ask whether we all saw it in front of us, and we all saw it in front of us. "What things that tower has seen! That tower saw Napoleon's soldiers. It saw Hitler's soldiers. It saw Anne Frank." (The tower had seen oppression, he told us, imprisonment, and I felt that he was thinking not just about the town's history, but about his own history, as well.) "And all kinds of storms have blown over this city, but that tower keeps standing there. It already stood there before I came along, and it'll still be there when I'm gone. My grandfather saw it. My father saw it. And now I'm here. And I go in that church, and I know: This is mine." And, after a silence, "Yeah, well, what I'm saying is probably pretty foolish."

"That's not foolish at all. I think it's very beautiful. What you're saying is said in almost the exact same way in the psalms. You're saying: 'O God, you are my rock, my help in ages past, my refuge from generation to generation, my shelter from the stormy blast, and my eternal home.' That's what you're saying."

The man looked at me, at first unbelievingly and then gratefully. "I should have been a minister," he said.

★ ★ ★

More and more I notice that people who have difficulty thinking abstractly, or who think that they are just simple souls, talk with me about the church and the tower if they want to say something about their faith or about God. Mostly they apologize for starting with mere stones and a building when I ask about their faith, but I'm quick to say that we can only talk about God in images anyway, and one image is no worse than another.

★ ★ ★

A boy had told me about all kinds of doubts, but he wanted to be confirmed anyway.

"You think you're ready for it?"

"Yes," he said. "It's really just like the Wester. It's in constant need of repair. But when I see those arches and pillars, then I think, Well it seems to be holding up OK, it doesn't seem to be about to tumble down, even though it's built on cowhides."

★ ★ ★

The loveliest song about the Wester is by that old Jewish singer Louis Davids:

O lovely old gray tower,
You've stood there many years.
And when I walk along the streets
Your presence calms my fears.
If only you could tell us
All that you've seen and heard,

The stories you could tell us!
But you never say a word.

O lovely old gray tower,
High in the sky so blue,
I dedicate my singing,
My laughs, my sighs, to you.
You know our deepest secrets,
Our woes, each laugh, each frown.
But you just play your bell songs
While silently looking down.

O wonderful, proud tower
I'm full of joy and pride
Whene'er the golden sunlight
Strikes your western side.
And when comes my last hour,
And all my powers flee,
Let them put my bed by the window,
So it's you, old tower, I'll see.

It seems clear to me that in this song of Davids the tower is a symbol for God, and so the question arises whether in heaven it's not just God but also the Wester Tower we'll see. On Sunday afternoons in the tavern we sing about that mystery:

Could another Jordaan in heaven be found
Just like in my old Amsterdam?
Will, high in the clouds, a tower clock sound
Like the Wester in Amsterdam?

Nobody in De Twee Zwaantjes realizes that the book of Revelation has already said no to that question, and that there will be no temple in the Holy City, heaven's Jerusalem, but in the café we keep hoping, for surely it can't be God's intention that up there we'll be worse off than we are here.

But since no one on earth in heaven has been,
The answer to that remains to be seen.

That's a song by Johnny Jordaan, our equivalent of Glen Campbell. He himself came to bring me the words.

Johnny and I talked about what the church and the tower mean to people around here.

se

"You have to swear to me that you'll never make a rug market out of it," Johnny said. "That's what happened to the Church of the Sower, over on the Rose Canal. I used to be a server at Mass there. Recently I went by to take a look at it for a minute. Nothing but rolls of carpet. I just had to whimper when I saw it. The Wester has to remain a church, y'hear. A church for everybody. You see it everywhere. Everywhere you walk you see it. I always have to look up at it for a moment. It's such a beautiful tower. I've always sung about it. Right from the heart, 'cause I mean what I sing. It's just as if that tower has a voice and is saying something."

I asked Johnny if I could read something to him.

"Of course," he said.

And I read:

Thou hast searched me and known me!
Thou knowest when I sit down and when I rise up;
Thou discernest my thoughts from afar . . .
and art acquainted with all my ways.
Thou dost beset me behind and before,
and layest thy hand upon me. (RSV)

"Yes, that's it, that's exactly it," said Johnny.

"It's a psalm," I said. "A psalm about God."

"Makes no difference," said Johnny.

We thought about that for a minute. Then my eye fell on the inscription of the psalm.

It read, "A Song of David."